WHEN CANCER CAME KNOCKING

How One Family Answered

Reverend Stephen Garrett

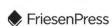 FriesenPress

Suite 300 - 990 Fort St
Victoria, BC, V8V 3K2
Canada

www.friesenpress.com

ISBN
978-1-5255-4339-5 (Hardcover)
978-1-5255-4340-1 (Paperback)
978-1-5255-4341-8 (eBook)

1. HEALTH & FITNESS, DISEASES, CANCER

Distributed to the trade by The Ingram Book Company

TABLE OF CONTENTS

DEDICATION

Peter's journey with cancer began in **February 2009** in Whitehorse, Yukon, with his first diagnosis, followed by his first treatment in **July of 2009**, and ended with his death on **September 17, 2015,** in the Butterfly Room of the Creston Hospital. It was our hope that he would have a while longer on this planet and with us so he could contribute some of his Irish humor to this book. With deep regret, his contributions will be limited to stories, texts, and emails.

It is to Peter Eric Garrett, his life and his death, that this book is dedicated.

INTRODUCTION

IN THE GRASP OF CANCER

I decided to write this book about four years ago, a year before my dear brother Peter died. Our family had been walking with cancer for five years already, and despite the challenges the disease brought to our doorstep, we had grown as individuals and as a family. Each in our own way, we were learning to love more deeply, to be more compassionate, to be even more grateful, and we were all learning how to live every day more fully.

Yes, in spite of cancer—the uninvited guest—showing up on our doorstep, our family learned how to navigate the many challenges and ups and downs of the crazy ride it took us on. We learned how to work with the medical system, as broken as it is; the cancer care system, as complex as it is; and our own family system, as crazy as it is. I thought it might be helpful to you, the reader, to learn of our story and experience it so it may make your journey with cancer less difficult to walk.

Each chapter features a "Different Perspectives" section that will illustrate how various people witnessing the same journey with cancer responded in their unique ways. It is important to know that we all react differently to the same dying and death process. It depends on our relationship with the one who is fighting for their life, coupled with our own personal relationship with death. I have asked two nurses to contribute to each chapter to let you know that even within the same system, each healthcare provider has their own personal response to the same death.

Each of the individuals has written his or her contribution. I have left them unedited in order that you can see clearly their unique responses to the challenges faced by Peter, and challenges they faced in their process of witnessing his walk with cancer.

You will also find throughout these chapters pieces of emails and text content that illustrate what is going on between the lines. These excerpts are real and often raw. They show the underbelly of what goes on when we walk the cancer path with chemotherapy, radiation, and modern medicine.

The Key Characters

The Late Peter Eric Garrett
About Peter (in his own words)

I was born in 1954, the fourth of five children, in Montreal just before the start of the Canadiens string of five consecutive Stanley Cups (still a record more than fifty years later). Sports were a strong theme growing up in our household. My brother and I were always involved in sports, hockey being the main one. Montreal brought that out in people back then. I am a father of three boys, an ex-husband, and a current husband. I work for the Canadian Government, and have been a laborer and lawyer, amongst other things. I never smoked, I drank sparingly, have eaten well, and led as good a life as I knew how.

Stephen Lloyd Garrett, Peter's elder brother
About Stephen

I was born in 1949, the first of five kids. I loved the Montreal Canadiens, and playing any kind of sports. I didn't really like school; I was shy and started dating in my late teens. I did the investment-banking thing for twenty-three years, social work for a decade, workshop facilitation for ten years, and finally discovered my true passion, dying and death education, which I have been pursuing passionately for the past seven years. I have a great wife and two amazing cats. I still love the Montreal Canadiens. I enjoy my work, gardening, and life in general. I am an Interfaith Minister.

April Garrett, Peter's wife
About April

April is a certified Reiki Master/Teacher in the Usui Shiki Ryoho Tradition, Karuna® Reiki Master and Lightarian™ Reiki Master, and holds a Basic Counselling Skills Certificate. She is also a certified Hawaiian Huna Kane™ Practitioner. April is currently working toward certification in Clinical Hypnotherapy. She has extensive experience facilitating workshops, classes, and support groups, as well as practical and experiential training in Transformational Breath Work Therapy and Shamanic Counseling, and individual spiritual development counseling. She opened the doors to House of Healing Light as a natural progression on her spiritual path in service to others. She is also a Licensed Practical Nurse.

Yvonne Heath, Nurse, Author, and Speaker
About Yvonne

I enjoyed "meeting" Peter, and felt myself wishing we had met. I wondered what I would have said to him along this journey. The nurse I was for twenty-seven years would have been compassionate, caring, and may have even made him laugh a time or two. I think I'm pretty funny! I would have tried diplomatically to encourage Peter to seek out the truth about treatment and prognosis. But I realize, looking back, that I was personally and professionally ill-prepared for grief, death, and dying. I realize that most of us are—yes, including doctors and nurses. So how could we help those facing the battle of their life to be prepared to face grief and possibly death?

Connie Jorsvik, Nurse and Patient Advocate
About Connie

I met Stephen as he was supporting Peter through the last months of his life. Stephen received his strength by helping others through their life-end journeys and their families understand the dying process. Stephen felt that Peter had not been given the complete picture of what to expect as he moved through treatments that caused so much additional pain and weakness. It was my pleasure to get to know Stephen during that time.

I have never feared death for others or myself. I was introduced to death early and intimately as a child, and my parents never hid me from it. Throughout my nursing career I was with countless patients as they passed through this life and onto the next. I had so many experiences that left me with no doubt there is a next life.

I am now a patient advocate and healthcare navigator and I teach Advanced Care Planning.

Marjorie Anne Garrett, Peter's Mom
About Marge

Marge was born May 21, 1928, in Toronto, Ontario. She married William Lloyd Garrett in 1948, had five kids, and raised them all as a stay-at-home mother. Later in life, she worked as a secretary for Sheppard Lodge Home for the Aged for ten years and volunteered for Hill House Hospice in Richmond Hill, Ontario, a privately run five room hospice, for another five years. Now eighty-nine years young, she lives in London, Ontario, with her daughter Carrie.

Mother dearest is a little on the blind side and not so efficient with things digital. Her contribution is in the form of an interview and transcribed by the author, her eldest son—me.

Caroline Norma Garrett, Peter's sister
About Carrie

Carrie is currently a Personal Support Worker. She has a couple of adult children from her first marriage. She lives in a fine home in London, Ontario, with her partner Charles, her mom, dogs Johnson and Angel, and two cats Hankie and Trixie. She is dedicated to serving our senior citizens to ensure they have the best quality of life they can. "I am all about advocating for seniors to ensure they have a peaceful, graceful, and as loving a life and a death as possible." She says with a big heart and a wide smile. Carrie worked in the retirement / assisted living industry.

In Summary

The unique written contribution of each person, their individual relationship with Peter, and their own beliefs and understanding around their ultimate death were all brought to bear during Peter's dying. Even as we each write for this book, we are all at different places in our own journey with the grief related to the death of our dear loved one. This speaks volumes to the art form that great hospice care is really all about.

When you read these Different Perspectives, notice how each one is unlike the ones before or after. The emotions, the reactions, how they write, and what they say may have some similar aspects, but the communication is uniquely theirs. Recognizing this will help you understand your own family dynamics when death comes knocking. You will be much more able to notice and accept all the different ways your family members grieve. It will create space for each person to let go their way and not have to behave like everyone else. It can be a little messy, but very much alive, real, human, and healing.

When It All Began

It all started just over nine years ago with Peter's first cancer diagnosis. It has been a long and winding road ever since. The first part of Peter's epic journey with cancer was captured in my book *When Death Speaks – Listen, Learn, and Love*. I include Peter's section here so you new readers can catch up with the early history of his walk with cancer.

My brother had faced cancer twice in the past couple of years and it was extremely challenging for him, not only physically but also mentally, emotionally, and spiritually. The beauty of it all, though, has been the growing relationship between the two of us and amongst our entire family. We are all much closer now that we ever have been. What a gift in spite of the challenges!

When I began writing *When Death Speaks*, I thought of Peter's journey with cancer and imagined it would be a helpful and inspiring story for you, the reader. I called Peter and asked him if he would consider writing a piece for this book. He thought it over, taking his time to make sure is was the right choice for him, and the right thing for the book. He said yes, so here is his contribution with only a few edits—after all, an older brother has some earned rights!

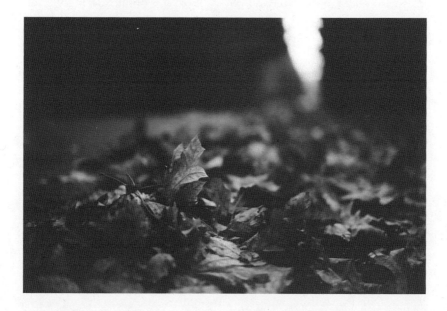

When my brother asked me to write a chapter for his new book, I asked him why. He said that he thought my 'near-death' experience (as he called it) might help others. When I asked him how long, he said between 2,000 to 3,000 words. Seriously? First of all, I'm Irish. Second, I used to be a lawyer (but it's okay—I saw the light and got out early). Now he wants me to use only 3,000 words? I suppose in some alternate universe that could happen. However, the sesquipedalian gene runs strong in my family. So, with absolutely no apologies to Stephen, here goes.

I was born in 1954, the fourth of five children, in Montreal just before the start of the Canadiens string of five consecutive Stanley Cups (still a record more than fifty years later). Sports were a strong theme growing up in our household. My brother and I were always involved in sports, hockey being the main one. Montreal brought that out in people back then. I am a father of three boys, an ex-husband, and a current husband. I work for the Canadian Government, and have been a laborer and lawyer, amongst other things. I never smoked, I drank sparingly, have eaten well, and led as good a life as I knew how. I won't bore you with all the other mundane historical pieces of my life, as they all somehow become much less important given the story I am about to share with you. With this unsatisfyingly short synopsis of my life, let's begin the part Stephen wants me to get to.

It was October 2008 and time for my annual physical. Towards the end, I pointed out a lump in my right groin and asked my family physician to check it out, explaining that I had had a similar one on my left groin about fifteen years earlier and it had turned out to be a benign fat deposit. I wasn't at all concerned this time as I assumed it would be the same kind of thing. However, the doctor was concerned and suggested that it was likely cancerous, and that I should consult the surgeon at the hospital. I was skeptical. The two lumps, to my mind (me being such a great medical specialist and all), looked the same. The previous one had been excised and sent for testing and came back as benign. Accordingly, I remained unconcerned.

Fast-forward to February 2009 and my meeting with the surgeon at Whitehorse General Hospital. He told me that he was 99% certain that I had cancer. Okay, that got my attention. The staff at the hospital told me there was an opening the next day for a biopsy, as a patient had just cancelled an appointment. Otherwise, there would be a four- to six-month wait. I told them that didn't work for me because I had to do a presentation the following day, so they put me on a wait list.

However, on the way back to the office, something unexpected happened. Halfway up the Two Mile Hill, I started crying and said aloud, 'I don't want to die.' I have never been overly comfortable with emotions, so this was a bit disconcerting. It was also good to realize that at the deepest level of my being, I was choosing life. I called the hospital as soon as I got back to the office and booked the available appointment for the biopsy. It took an extremely long month to get the results back.

The day finally arrived. The call was holding for me.

Unfortunately, the doctor had a thick accent and I was unable to understand what he was saying. I called the medical office and asked them to have someone I could understand call me. After all, this was important to me and I wanted a degree of certainty about the results. Five minutes later, I received another call, and to my surprise, it was the same doctor. After several minutes of not understanding anything he was saying, I finally said, 'Doctor, I am sorry but I cannot understand what you are saying. It may be the phone connection, it may be me, but I need to be clear about the results. So, I am going to ask you a question and I want you to respond with a single word only. Do I have cancer?'

The answer was crystal clear: 'YES!'

That set into motion a series of tests to determine the extent and location of the cancer, culminating with a very strong 'suggestion' from my oncologist that I immediately undergo radiation therapy. He explained the cancer was neither widespread nor aggressive. He also said that I was young and healthy (which immediately catapulted him to the top of my Christmas card list), and that this was the ideal time to 'stop this thing'— this thing being Non-Hodgkin's Lymphoma.

At the time, I was tele-working from my home in the Kootenays. The closest cancer clinic in British Columbia was in Kelowna, a half-day's drive from my place. The arrangements were made. I was to begin radiation treatments in four months—July 2009.

I felt optimistic and got on with my life while awaiting the treatments. I arrived the Sunday before they were to start and checked into the cancer care lodge immediately adjacent to the cancer clinic. The lodge was a godsend, as hotels in the Okanagan in the middle of summer can be pricey. The lodge was not only affordably priced, but it also included all meals and had a nurse on staff. In addition, it had an incredible group of volunteers, without whom the lodge could not function.

I checked in and got unpacked in my half of the room (turns out I was to have a roommate), and then went down to the cafeteria for dinner. I grabbed a tray and headed towards the line-up, but stopped halfway there, frozen in place.

It finally hit me that my cancer was real. I was going to get my first radiation treatment the next morning. All this time, I thought that I had been handling things well. More likely, I had been in denial. I could not move. I felt overwhelmed, terrified, and alone.

A hand gently touched my shoulder. I heard a voice asking me if I was okay. It was one of the other residents of the lodge. Slowly I turned to her and said, 'It just hit me that this is all real.' I didn't elaborate, nor did I have to. The compassionate look on her face told me she understood exactly what I was saying. She asked me if I would like to join her and her friends at their table. I gratefully accepted. She stayed with me while I went through the line-up for dinner and then walked me back to the table.

Though seemingly a little thing, it meant so much to me (and still does) that she recognized what I was going through and chose to help me. The group was entirely composed of women. We did the round of introductions and they quickly returned to their conversation. They discussed a variety of things, including their upcoming treatments, but the tone was surprisingly upbeat and positive. I heard nothing along the lines of 'poor me' or 'why is this happening to me?' It turns out that this was common for almost all of the residents of the lodge.

It was not that they didn't realize the seriousness of the situation, but that they chose not to give away their power to it. They all chose to make the best of it. During the entire length of my stay, I met only two people who focused on the negative. I was inspired by those who chose the positive route so much so that I chose that road too!

Now, this is not to say that they didn't have bad days; we all did. It was just that, overall, we chose life and to focus on the positive aspects of being alive. I remained part of the group for my entire stay at the clinic.

One night in the dessert line-up, I noticed one of the women filling her plate with pie, ice cream, and other sweet things. I didn't say anything, but must have raised my eyebrows in surprise. She turned to me and said, 'Peter, I have cancer. No one is going to tell me what I can or can't eat!' I laughed, somewhat embarrassed, and asked if I could borrow that line from time to time. When she left on her 'Emancipation Day' a couple of weeks later, I gave her a gift from the local Winners store: an ice cream serving set.

I started my treatments on a Monday morning, and they were to be done daily, Monday to Friday. Thankfully, I got weekends off. The first day, they made three small tattoos on my body so that they could triangulate the machine in order to radiate exactly the same area each time. Trying more to quell my nervousness than to make them laugh, I asked whether I could choose my tattoo pattern. They said, 'No, it is really only three small dots.' I asked if I could choose a color only to be rebuffed again.

After they tattooed me, I had my first treatment. The machine was enormous and looked like something straight out of a Star Wars movie. Most of the session was spent lining up the machine with the tattoos. The actual radiation portion seemed rather brief. I actually felt nothing during the treatments themselves. I discovered that the side effects would kick in later. This became the central part of each day, in relation to which all other things were secondary.

There were set meal times and, except for really bad days, I rarely missed a meal. I usually sat with the group I had met on the first night. The radiation technicians were excellent, and were both professional and friendly. They were also a great source of help in me understanding what my body was going through. They would recommend things for the simpler side effects, and referred me to my oncologist for the more complex affects.

On weekends, I would drive the five-and-a-half hours home to Wynell to reconnect with my wife, April. Fortunately, one of the other residents, Bev, had given me a gel seat to make the drive more endurable (at least as far as one of the side effects was concerned). The two days always passed far too quickly, and by Sunday night, I was back at the lodge in Kelowna.

During my time at the clinic, I began to consider the possibility that this cancer might have happened for a reason, so I began to explore what that might be. The cancer clinic had arranged weekly meditation sessions, and one of the women at my table, Darla, had asked me whether I would like to attend. I readily agreed and quite enjoyed them.

After doing a lot of reading and meditation, I concluded that I had spent far too much of my life being a Type A personality, a perfectionist, and a bit of a workaholic. I was reminded about a cliché: *nobody on their deathbed ever says: 'I wish I had spent more time in the office'.* I realized this had to change. I also felt that I had done a lot for others but had failed to honor myself. It was not that I regretted having done things for others, but that I regretted not including myself in that process. I promised myself this would change.

Soon enough, my own Emancipation Day arrived. I said my goodbyes and made my way home to await the results of my final tests. It took quite some time. Three months passed before my oncologist advised me that I was in remission. Obviously, I was relieved. April and I celebrated.

However, I did not bounce back the way I felt I should have. I know my body fairly well, and it seemed not to be responding to my newly diagnosed healthy state. I checked with the doctors but they suggested that I give it more time; that recovery can be a slow process.

Slightly more than a year after my treatments had ended, I went to a local naturopath in Whitehorse, where I was now living. I told her what I had been through and what I was currently experiencing. She gave me some supplements to help with the aftermath of cancer treatments. These tablets made the side of my neck swell up so I decided on my own to discontinue them.

At my next appointment, I asked her why that happened. She was unsure and said she would research it for me. About a month later, she had been unable to discover anything about this side effect and simply suggested a different kind of supplement. I tried them, only to have the same result—my neck swelled up again.

Curious, I asked whether that might be because the supplements had detected cancer cells and were trying to fight them instead of simply helping me to recover from the treatments. She thought that might be a possibility, so I immediately booked an appointment with my family doctor. One look at my neck, and knowing my medical history, she immediately scheduled another series of cancer tests for me. I was back in the hospital having blood work, x-rays, ultrasound and, of course, the infamous CT scan.

Again, the waiting game.

Hoping against hope that the results would show me to be cancer-free, I waited for the call. The response was fairly quick this time, a matter of weeks.

Not only had the non-Hodgkin's Lymphoma returned but another cancer had been detected: Hodgkin's Lymphoma, both in my neck. My oncologist told me not to worry. Hodgkin's Lymphoma was better than Non-Hodgkin's, and he set up chemotherapy treatments right away. I advised him that I wanted some time to think about it first and consider other options. In spite of my delay tactics, I received a call from the cancer centre in the Whitehorse General Hospital a week or so later wanting to schedule my treatments.

When I advised the nurse that I wanted to explore other options, she enquired as to what those might be. When I asked why, she seemed concerned and responded, 'Did you know that Hodgkin's Lymphoma, if left untreated, is fatal?' I was shocked, as my oncologist had not seen fit to share that particular fact with me. Suddenly, I did not have the time I had thought to pursue naturopathic avenues of treatment.

'Fatal' was not something I wanted to mess with. Once again, I was face to face with cancer.

However, in spite of the attention grabbing 'fatal' aspect, the prognosis for Hodgkin's Lymphoma is quite good, with a survival percentage in the 80–90% range. I was not dreading the chemotherapy, but was not doing cartwheels about it either. Somewhat reluctantly, I agreed to start the treatments right away.

Fortunately, the Whitehorse General Hospital is set up to administer chemotherapy, so I was spared the ordeal of having to fly south to a major centre for the treatments. I began the four-month regimen of chemo treatments, one every two weeks. I had foolishly thought at the beginning, 'Once every two weeks, how hard can that be?' My radiation treatments had been daily, so I figured that this shouldn't be too tough.

That line of thinking came to an abrupt end with the first treatment.

I experienced every one of the possible side effects I was warned about, and some they didn't—the latter including hiccoughs, the extended play version, and an accelerated heart rate that lasted days at a time. I had chosen to make my battle with cancer more widely known this time, primarily for the reason that I was working in an office in Whitehorse. Being a small town, word travels quickly, and I assumed that once my hair started falling out (more quickly than my advancing years was causing), people would figure it out. Letting people know turned out to be the best thing I could have done.

The more difficult part was letting my children know. They had been quite worried the first time around and I was not looking forward to telling them I was having a second series of cancer treatments. I needn't have worried so much, as they are great kids. Darren even offered to move north and look after me—a sincere and much appreciated offer. I was overwhelmed by the amount of support I was to receive.

Aside from Darren, a number of other people offered to move in with me and help me out during the course of my treatments. I chose not to accept any of these generous and loving offers, and I was grateful for the compassion behind them.

I am also blessed with many great friends in Whitehorse, and they were incredibly supportive.

At first, I found this difficult to accept, and I had to figure out why that was. Turns out I like to be the one doing the giving and not so much the one accepting. Learning from my first experience with cancer, I meditated about this, and the answer I got was twofold:

1. *It is time to let go of the resistance and allow yourself to accept good things into your life (it ties in well with the concept of honoring myself) and,*

2. *Other people do care and want to help, so why would I want to deny them that opportunity?*

Needless to say, I chose to accept the support, and it was a wise decision. On my worst days, when white cell counts were extremely low and it was not healthy for me to be out in public, friends would shop for me. They would leave the grocery bags on my doorstep and ring the bell, staying a safe distance away so as not to run the risk of spreading their germs. Other friends cooked meals in for me; soup was much appreciated on days when my tongue and throat were swollen and sore.

People at work who I had not known that well offered to help me get through this ordeal. I was blown away by all this kind support. It showed me, up close and personal, people are at the core of their beings amazing and compassionate. It brought me to tears. My older brother (the one compiling this book) called me regularly to check in on me, giving me what loving support he could from a couple of thousand miles away. This was a huge gift, as he and I have never had a close relationship up until this point. It was an unexpected and much appreciated silver lining.

A second gift was my sons helping me learn about the world of texting, and we stayed in touch frequently through that medium. This is not to say that the experience was all New Age Love and Enlightenment—not by a long shot. There were days when the pain was extremely intense, and the Cancer Clinic only wanted me to take acetaminophen so as not to interfere with what the chemo was doing. I both understood and supported their reasoning intellectually. However, on a purely physical level, it was an entirely different matter. The acetaminophen did absolutely nothing for my pain.

It felt as though all my joints were on fire. I could not sleep and I was unable to find a pain-free position. I tried every piece of furniture in the house, and even the floor, but nothing supported my quest for sleep. Some days, my painful sleeplessness was combined with pain and swelling in my throat and tongue, so much so that I could barely swallow even soft things. I just wanted to curl up in a ball and die.

I tried to focus on the big picture and remind myself that this was a temporary period that would end soon enough, and that I would, in all likelihood, recover. By the end of each two-week period, I would inevitably start to feel better and be 'ready' just in time to start the cycle of chemo. I went to work as often as I could. I do like my job and the great people there. It was also therapeutic; being at work, and focusing on tasks there, took my mind off my personal situation for a while.

Was chemotherapy a challenging experience to go through? Absolutely.

Did my potential death force me to the wall? Undoubtedly. Am I going to tell you that I came close to death, saw the light, and my late sister, Jody?

No, but I came very close.

My experience with cancer showed me that both life and people are very special, and that I will never know when either could be taken from me. I am resolved to do my best to enjoy and appreciate my own life, my family, and friends. I made new friends and new discoveries about myself, both helping my life be more fulfilling and joyful than it was.

Am I out of the woods? No. The Hodgkin's Lymphoma is in remission, but the non-Hodgkin's Lymphoma is still with me. It is not widespread and will be monitored regularly. To me, this is fairly minor in the grand scheme of things.

What's next? Well, truth be told, I kinda like my brother's new motto in his career as what I am calling a 'Life or Death Coach':

Create a Life Worth Dying For and a Death Worth Living For! I am going to get started on just that!

Catching Up

It is **March 23, 2010,** and though life seems pretty normal, it really isn't. The content of this email would suggest so, yet all the while cancer is lurking just below the surface in remission.

> On 2010-03-22, at 7:42 PM, Peter Garrett wrote:

>> yes - I am still trying to figure out what I want to be when I grow up. Let me know how that process goes.

>> I decided to buy the townhouse and paid the full deposit today. Closing date of November 30 - hopefully the can-buck stays strong until the fall so Harper (oops) Carney will keep rates where they are.

>> Have a great week!
>> Peter

Read between the lines written on **March 25th of 2013.**

> On 2013-03-25, at 7:21 PM, Peter Garrett wrote:

>> Thanks, bro. The news today from my Oncologist was not bad. The blood tests show the cancer is present - no surprise there. BUT he feels it is not progressing at an alarming rate, which is a big change from the

prognosis last fall. Evidently, some of the stuff I am doing must be working. He needs to get the rest of the test results (a week or so) but he said he would be surprised if they were different than those we discussed today.

Under the circumstances, it was a good meeting. He will await my decision but I told him that, given there appears to be no immediate threat, I would likely continue to pursue alternative protocols rather than subject myself to chemo/radiation again.

Now to decide what that next protocol will be...

Peter

The saga continues well into **August of 2014.**

On Aug 5, 2014, at 7:45 PM, Peter Garrett <petergarrett2004@yahoo.ca> wrote:

Hey, guys.

It has been a challenge but I may have found the clinic I will take my treatments at:

http://www.germancancerclinics.com/hyperthermia-centre

They have everything I have been seeking and then some. And, if you believe in "trusting your gut", this place feels right as well. And I get to be in Germany!

Needless to say, it will be pricey—that is the challenge with pretty much all private clinics. However, I am lucky to have some great friends up here and they told me (whether I liked it or not) that they would do a bunch of fundraisers for me. They are amazing.

That also got me thinking that, seeing as Darren was willing to wear a Tom Brady jersey anyway, he could contact the team for me and schmooze some money out of them... :-)

So, I see my Naturopathic doctor Wednesday to go over all my results and my current plan. She has been great over the past couple of years and I value her opinion. Then April and I will have a good yak tomorrow night and if all the lights are still green, I will make the arrangements.

For the first time in a week and a half, I am getting excited.

I will keep you posted.

Have a great week!
Peter

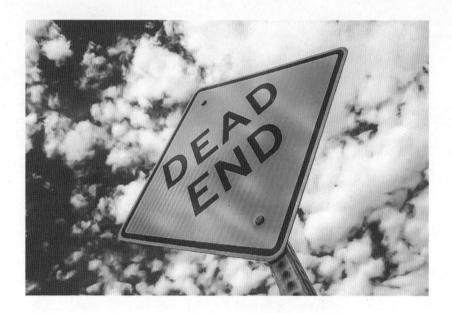

All of a sudden, it is **May 10, 2015,** six years into Peter's journey with cancer. I am picking him up at the Vancouver International Airport and dropping him off at the Cancer Care Cottage at 10th and Ash in downtown Vancouver. We got him comfortably tucked into his room as he prepared for the fight of his life.

Fast forward to **July 29, 2015,** after six plus years of radiation, chemotherapy, and stem cell treatments. I asked my dear brother Peter if he was feeling up to some writing for this my second book on dying, death, and grief.

Here is his response via text:

> "I will have to get back to you. This recovery thing is
> harder than I expected. Exhausted, in a lot of pain still
> and emotionally drained. I know things will improve
> but I am feeling overwhelmed and useless at the
> moment. Do not need a pep talk. I understand things

quite well in my noggin. Just need to be patient and keep putting one foot in front of another. And give my body the rest it needs."

I found myself wondering if he would have made a different choice had he had more 'real' information on how his recovery would go and what the quality of his life would be.

"Would you do this again, Peter, knowing what you know now?" I asked.

"No," was his only reply.

The chapters of this book are all about distinctly different looks at the same cancer journey: my brother Peter's intimate and subjective view as only he could experience it, along with the views of those of us around him that are somewhat more removed or a little less subjective. My intention is that you the reader get to see the innermost intimate pieces of this challenging yet wondrous adventure and that those pieces, the 'stuff' no one really wants to talk about, get exposed to the light of the day for all to learn and grow by.

CHAPTER ONE

WHAT HAPPENED, I WAS IN REMISSION, WASN'T I?

Both Peter and April felt the profound relief that comes with hearing cancer is in remission. All of us were breathing much easier knowing Peter's cancer had been beaten back. From his kids, his mom, his work associates, me, and everyone in between, there was a collective yahoo and a sigh of relief. Life could get back to 'normal'; dying and death had been averted, at least temporarily.

The respite was short lived for me, yet in Peter's world of walking with cancer, two years was much like a lifetime. Cancer had reared its head again. It had morphed, migrated, and found its way into his bone structure, continuing its unrelenting march through Peter's body almost at will, even with all that the medical system had thrown at it so far.

The Summer of 2014 – Not Again!

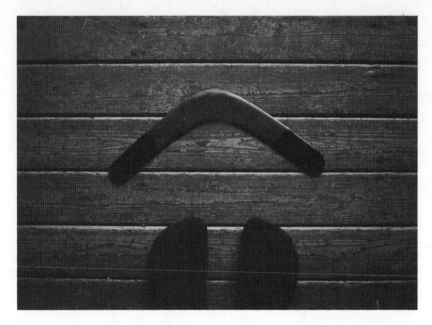

Things started to go sideways. Peter's body began to show signs that cancer was knocking again. There was a lump here and a lump there and tenderness and pain was developing. The cancer had migrated to Peter's upper body and now he was looking at Hodgkin and Non-Hodgkin's lymphoma in his neck, underarm, shoulder, and chest.

"How the hell do I tell my family that the battle is back on?" he must have thought.

Peter was reluctant to speak to his family and friends, with the exception of April and myself. Though I didn't agree with his lack of enthusiasm to speak out about the return of cancer, I totally understood it. Stepping back into the ring with the Michael Tyson of cancer was not an appealing thought for Peter particularly, never mind for the rest of us. He didn't want to alarm any of us by bring the cancer card back on the table, where we would all have to face it. Cancer would again become the topic of too many conversations.

No matter how he would phrase it, what words he would chose, what tone of voice he would use, there was no doubt the alarm bells would ring in his family life, his work life, and his social life.

On Aug 17, 2014, at 7:25 PM, Peter Garrett <petergar-rett2004@yahoo.ca> wrote:

Hey guys.

Things are starting to move quickly...

For the past week, I have had very little sleep due to the pain the cancer is causing in various parts of my body. Then last Thursday night, there was such intense pain in my chest that I felt like I was having a heart attack. After I talked myself out of going to Emergency (they would have been disappointed I didn't arrive with cookies), I palpated the area and found that there was pain in the ribs and some neuropathy in the muscle tissue. Clearly, the cancer was targeting a new area.

It underscored that perhaps Dr. Villa (my oncologist) was correct about there being a short window of opportunity and waiting another 2 1/2 weeks to get into an alternative clinic was probably now the poorer choice. Who knows how much more damage the cancer might cause by then? I might not even be able to travel.

Sooo, I have reluctantly agreed to undergo the chemo protocol that deals with diffuse large cell B lymphoma. I advised the Chemo Nurse on Friday and she has me booked to see Dr. Sally McDonald (she is the doctor who supervises all things chemo at the hospital) Tuesday morning at 10:00. Then I will start chemo (the first one is a two day extravaganza) either W/TH or TH/F next week (i.e. either the 20/21 or the 21/22). After that once every three weeks for a total of 4 1/2 months.

As this part of it has happened rather suddenly, I plan to be at work for the first week or so (or longer) depending on the severity of the side effects. In all likelihood, I will be submitting a request for long-term disability sometime soon.

After making the decision, I felt a sense of relief and believe that this is the best decision under the circumstances. And out of respect for my mom, I have requested a prescription for marijuana (Carrie - make sure you tell her that!).

What a crazy ride this past few weeks have been!

Love you all,
Peter

Death this time seemed even closer than before, and the loss of Peter felt even more pressing. This louder knocking on the door triggered some very human reactions in all of us:

Combativeness - Hope / Denial - Fear - Anger
Confusion – Bargaining – Depression
Sadness - Discomfort

- "We'll beat this damn thing!"

- "The German's have had great success with targeted chemo and stem cell

- treatments. I am sure it will work for Peter"

- "It can't be happening to Peter again."

- "No way! Not again!"

- "Maybe they mixed up the charts by mistake."

- "Oh please anyone but Peter. He doesn't deserve this."

- "Can't it all be a bad mistake?"

- "I just don't want to talk about it."

- "Not again!"

- "How can God let this happen?"

No matter what the reactions were, there was no arguing: cancer was ferociously back and we all had to face its music. It seemed as if we vaulted from remission to battle without any warning at all. Cancer didn't care though about any of our worries, concerns, or prayers. It was back in the family. The uninvited and unwanted guest had returned.

Yes, we had to feel it all, notice our reactions, and find healthy ways to express ourselves. That is part of self-care and staying alive and present in the face of potential and probable death. We all simply had to get on with the reality of Peter's life. What are our next steps along this unique and challenging path? Round three began, as did chemotherapy and all its attendant nasty challenges.

Different Points of View
Peter - posthumously

Peter was deflated. He so wanted a 'normal' life back, a life he could live fully. Scared, frightened, concerned, alarmed, panicked, confused, frustrated, pissed off, and angry are other words that you could use to describe Peter's emotional state. He hid all this under a mask of optimistic stoicism, and only a few were invited to witness his innermost feelings.

He also didn't want to alarm his family, so he sheltered us all from the reality of his situation. He did his best to stay positive and focused on beating cancer. Sure, he had a chemo doctor, and Peter was his own spin-doctor, doing what he could to limit the impact round three would have on the rest of us. He was always able to put a positive twist on things.

His humorous stoicism, though noble and inspiring, was also problematic. Read the text below to see what I mean.

September 6, 2014 Sat Peter Garrett Text

"Hey Garrett Guys. Hope u r all having an amazing weekend. Back to the hair falling out stage so shaved it all off last night... just in time for winter. Ah, well good excuse to wear my Habs toques. Love ya. Peter."

April

The feelings of celebration and relief, albeit a brief sanctuary from what had become a surreal and unknown journey for both of us was over again. Then there was momentary panic: what does this mean now? I remember slipping into the familiar territory of feeling panic and then focusing again on being present for Peter. We talked openly about our feelings, the changes in our plans, and the necessary adjustments to being in a life together with cancer. I knew that Peter would die; when and how were the unknowns. How could we navigate through life, knowing that the horrible eventuality would occur, with the strength and conviction of spirit we both needed was the challenge? It was service of the highest order and I felt honored to be able to be by his side.

Stephen

My first reaction was "Not again!" I was pissed off that Peter had to deal with cancer a third time. Hadn't he gone through enough? I didn't wish it were happening to me in his place, I am not that selfless, I just wished it wasn't happening to him. Underneath my anger and upset lay a disturbing thought: "I don't think he is going to make it." Was this my way of preparing for the death of my brother, to sneak in this sort of thinking just in case? I kept shifting between being angry and pissed off and being deeply sad that this could be the end of Peter's life.

Upset though I was, I stayed in touch with Peter regularly and checked in often. I did my best to put him and his life first before launching into my questions about his health—a lesson Peter had taught me earlier on in this wild roller coaster ride with cancer. See the text below.

On 2013-03-22, at 6:53 AM, Peter Garrett wrote:

> "As for informing people, I will do that at the time things turn even more serious (i.e. if my oncologist advises that things have deteriorated and he feels there is no other option than immediate chemo). Once everyone knows, they treat you differently; all conversations focus on the cancer/your health; they look at you differently; many people avoid you because they can't deal with it, etc. Don't get me wrong, most people are coming from a place of caring and that is awesome, BUT the dynamics are immediately changed and it is very challenging to deal with. I have been down this path a couple of times now and I know how it works."

Yvonne

I can't even begin to imagine the relief and deep joy Peter and April experienced hearing the beautiful word "remission." It must feel like the second chance you were praying for, like it wasn't your time after all. I am glad for them, that they experienced that joy.

The downside is how much harder you must fall hearing the words "it's back" and feeling that deep disbelief. "Here we go again!" I feel such deep sadness, not knowing personally, but having been witness to, this one too many times, and knowing what this family endured again.

I can't help but wonder about this. In line with the rest of our death-phobic society, April and Peter were perhaps ill prepared for grief, death, and dying. They may not have faced their mortality when they were young and healthy. I wonder if in these two years of supposed remission, had they carved out time for "The Talk." I wonder if they had talked, planned, and prepared for life and the end of life, discussed their beliefs about life and death, and that living a full life has nothing to do with how long we are here. I wonder if they had structured their life in such a way that they could live without each other, and celebrated the time they were together, would the rest of their journey through cancer have been very different?

How would it have looked if society (i.e. health care professionals and everyone who touched their lives) were well-prepared for grief, death, and dying? Would April and Peter have been well supported in a decision not to fight the good fight to the bitter end? Would Peter's "humorous stoicism" and his need to soften the blow for those he loved not been necessary?

Connie

From my perspective as a nurse, it looks like the deeper conversations around Peter's health were missed. These deeper chats would have helped the family deal with the possibility of cancer returning, as is more common than not. Now was the time for the quality versus quantity talk. A familiar refrain I often heard was, "We beat it the first time so we'll beat it again."

Because some patients have first-hand experience with the chemo regime, as does the medical system, it can be easy to slip right back into the chemo and radiation treatment plan. Doctors feel comfortable in treatment, families feel hopeful that cancer can be beaten again, and we all miss the chance for a more meaningful and real conversation. The discomfort doctors feel about talking about dying and death, coupled with our own fear and denial of it, close the door to dialogue that could help families plan more effectively and with more realism.

I believe that planning for dying frees up emotional space for living.

Carrie

It seems like just yesterday I got the news that my brother Peter had non-Hodgkin's lymphoma. My initial reaction was "thank goodness it can be beat." It went into remission until another form of lymphatic cancer appeared, and was more aggressive. Damn it, I thought! Why does Peter have to go through this?!

That was just over six years ago now. Peter's battle with cancer was such an up and down, painful, and exhausting journey over all that time. I couldn't imagine what I would have done had it been me, and believe me, I wanted it to be me not him. I worried about Peter and his wife April every day. I wanted to be there for them both every second of the day, if I could. I felt like the universe had played a cruel trick on my brother, his wife, our family, and his friends. How dare he get cancer and possibly die! Damn the universe and its tricks!

That was the beginning of my grief for Peter's cancer battle.

Marge

"Mom, what was your first reaction when you learned of the return of Peter's cancer?" I asked.

"Oh no, not again!" Marge recalled. "This is the third time. Poor Pete."

"I tend to go on hold emotionally and wait for further developments and clarification of what's happening," Mom said. "I listened to what Peter had to say and his plans for alternative therapy and thought it was worthwhile."

"I had to stop and wait to see it through with him. I tried not to let Peter know of my worries. I chose to go through it with him day by day. I didn't want to add my emotions and worries to what he was already dealing with."

CHAPTER TWO

THE NEVER ENDING RESEARCH

Round three was successful but only on a temporary basis. The cancer returned within months and Peter battled on. I am not sure if it was fueled by denial and fear or a desire to live, but over the next four months, Peter and the rest of us began to search the Internet for possible treatments and alternatives to the more traditional ways our North American healthcare system fights cancer: radiation, chemotherapy, and surgery.

We searched high and low, especially Peter. His burning desire for five more years of life was a powerful motivator. We looked at naturopathic, allopathic, and combinations of both. We looked at herbal medicine, marijuana oil, joints, and unique potions I had never heard of before. I had lengthy discussions with a naturopathic oncologist friend of mine hoping for some inside information and a new treatment for cancer. Meditation practices, color and sound therapy, reiki, distant healing, chanting, drumming, and sacred ceremonies with shaman were all explored and many tired. Mexico, Germany, the Netherlands, Iceland, Bali, Peru, and India, amongst others, were all researched for their possible positive geographic impact on fighting Peter's cancer.

We narrowed our search down to Germany and a well-tested treatment regime called Targeted Chemotherapy. It combined the best of the allopathic system and the best of the naturopathic approach to treat the whole person. As we all honed in on this treatment plan, it looked like Peter was heading to Germany. At worst, he and April would have a great final vacation; at best, the cancer would go into remission again. We began to create a plan.

Luck, however, was not on our side, and our planning came to a screeching halt.

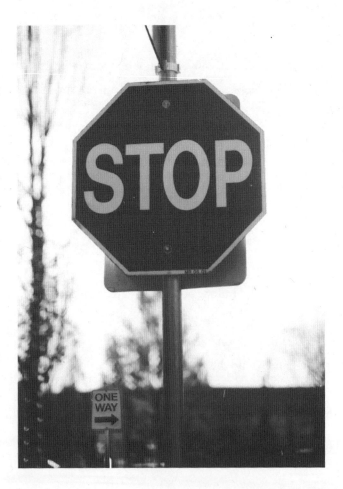

Peter's health needs became much more complex and urgent. All earlier plans around alternative treatment were shelved. Along with the cancer, his thrombosis team had noticed many more blood clots in his system. Travelling, especially flying and lengthy drives, were out of the question. His oncologist, the amazing Sally, as Peter often referred to her, and her team were extremely concerned about the aggressiveness of the cancer and its rapid growth. There was no time to experiment. This was serious. Peter was very concerned and frightened by the prospects.

He chose to take the medical system's advice. No Germany.

Our road trip from Whitehorse to Vancouver was nixed. Blood clots ruled out sitting for long periods. New plans were set, flights booked, and all of a sudden we were all systems go for more of the same: chemotherapy. His days were soon filled with intense scanning and prodding, an incalculable number of blood tests from veins nearly impossible to find, tubes inserted through his chest into his heart, and all manner of medical interventions. The plan included harvesting his own stem cells, putting the healthy ones on ice, and preparing his body for six more days of bombastic chemo, followed by a short recovery time, and then reintroducing his stem cells into the desert of his body.

Different Points of View
Peter - posthumously

Despite Peter's bravado, he was scared shitless. His cancer was unrelenting and seemingly undefeatable. He didn't really know what to do aside from react to the very nervous, almost panicked urgings of his medical team.

The urgency expressed by his doctors convinced him to go with the tried and true medical approach. He did so despite his earlier thoughts and feelings about the use of even more chemotherapy.

April

In some ways, it was easier knowing that all I had to do was love him. There was nothing really to do or say of a medical nature. I had done all the research, done the palliative training, and exhausted all the known approaches to this disease. All I could do now was be there for him, to let him talk if he needed, hold and be with him as he wanted, and to keep him focused on what was real and good within him and the world. That is who he was. It was like creating a bubble to hold everything, myself included, encompassing the feeling of peace, and his determined focus not to lose himself in the pain and confusion of learning from cancer. This is how he choose to view it.

Stephen

I was angry and sad all at the same time. I was angry that our road trip had been cancelled; it was going to be some great quality time with Peter and selfishly I resented it being taken away. I was sad too because I had had this sense that Peter wasn't going to make it for a few years now, and it looked like I was right. I was upset, mad actually, that Peter had chosen the chemo path again, against his own feelings and the urgings of his family. It seemed like Peter had succumbed to a marketing plan of sorts to get him to do yet another round of chemo. It was quantity over quality, and I didn't agree at all with his choice. It was HIS choice though, so I finally let my judgments go and jumped onto his page as best I could. He needed cheerleaders, not opponents. Most importantly, I stayed in close touch with Peter daily.

Yvonne

It would be wonderful to explore alternative therapies, not in desperation but with the idea, "let's do the best we can, and live life to the fullest in the process." And to be able to have heart to heart conversations, raw and honest, about how painful the quest for health against all odds is for the rest of us. If we could be okay with laughing, crying, pleading with each other, even having a good brawl, then maybe we could allow reality to play its part.

Were the doctors honest about Peter's prognosis? Did he truly understand that having gone through chemo twice, then to subject himself to stem cell transplant was a long shot at best? Were these doctors honest with themselves?

Connie

I'm a communications specialist and this was another opportunity lost. Doctors are stuck in their agenda of eradicating disease, but this was the moment to get real about the chances for recovery and what that would mean. The doctors may not have had to give definitive dates, definitive expectations of what would happen without the treatment, but they would have had a pretty good idea about the side effects and quality of life during the treatments.

It's been my experience (reinforced by research) that when given the option, patients pick quality over quantity every time.

Peter and his family were undergoing profound grief, not only due to the cancer, but because their dreams and hopes being crushed. Each person wanted extra time, a special trip, special conversations, and all of that had been taken away. No one felt they could say a word. The die had been cast and the new treatments would begin.

Carrie

As life tends to do, everything moved forward, along with Peter's cancer. I remember thinking, 'I wish he would stop taking treatments and just live out the rest of what life he has left with as much love, joy, laughter, and passion as he can.' But Peter had other plans, stubborn Irishman that he was! He tried the natural cancer treatments, and the traditional ones, along with pain meds such as morphine and natural pain meds like marijuana oil.

I cringed, I cried, I yelled, and I stamped my feet at the thought of all he and April were going through. I wanted it to be over, and for Peter to resume his everyday life as a cancer free man. The universe had other plans for my BB (Big Bother—the nickname I used to call him).

Peter made the decision to go through stem cell transplant therapy to kill nearly every good living cell in his body and then reintroduce his stem cells to create new healthy cells and destroy his cancer.

Marge

"Mom, how was it for you to hear that even more chemo was on the way?" I asked.

"Peter was only sixty and he still had a chance at a good life. He loved his wife April so much, and I guess he had to do it. If he were a single man he may have chosen differently," Marge said. "Peter was such a good researcher and so analytical that I trusted he was making the right decision for him."

"Were you worried?" I asked.

"No. I knew he was in April's good care and that he would work his way through it all. I knew Peter wasn't telling me the whole truth, in a way to protect me. I played the game in a way," Mother recalled. "In a way I think we all did."

CHAPTER THREE

LOTS OF HOPE AND
A STIFF UPPER LIP

With the decision made to proceed with this new intense targeted chemotherapy, we all had to let go of our own preferences for Peter and get on board the treatment regime he had chosen. I was personally deeply disappointed. I had been a strong advocate for a trip to Germany to take advantage of their more holistic approach to cancer. I was having a hard time getting my head around even more chemo, intensely more, given the already weakened state of Peter's body. Personally, I would not have made that choice, and yes, it's true I was not in Peter's shoes facing cancer again and the even stronger knock of death this time. It's easy for me to say.

Peter had made his selection and now I chose to line up with him and stand by his side, to be with him as he walked along this medical model pathway we each knew all too well. I knew that any further harping on my more naturopathic preferences would have been a bit on the abusive side and clearly not helpful, as Peter had made his decision. With a heavy heart, I set my preferences aside and sat my sorry ass down by his bed.

As quickly as the word got out about Peter's cancer, so too did the hopefulness. His friends were hopeful; his family, his kids, siblings, and our mom all jumped on the hope bandwagon. Everyone began to site the statistics from the German approach that was similar to the targeted chemo approach Peter had chosen here at home. The success rates were this, or that, on and on it went.

Now, I am not one of those hopeful sorts of fellows. I am more inclined to have faith and intention rather than hope, so I stayed away from the buzz of the statistics. Instead, I decided to have faith that Peter had made the right choice for himself. I held the firm intention that he heal and be well again while at the same time being pragmatic and plan for the worst just in case. It was a challenging balance.

I felt the need to be realistic. Having a background in finance and economics, I knew how simple it was to roll off successful results and make things 'look' a certain way. It is a numbers game. The business of cancer is no different and successful statistics keep the money flowing in, the financial donors happy that they are fighting a winning cause. These same success stats keep the patients coming too.

That being said, I needed to ask what success meant in this world of cancer treatments. It was darn near impossible to get clear information. What I did find was a muddle of statistics, numbers with no clear statement of what success meant or how it was measured. As it turned out, all the studies I could find measured success as length of life after treatment, meaning walking out of the hospital alive. None measured quality of life; only the quantity was researched.

Special Note:
Beware of the statistics; they are comforting to hang your
hope hat on, and they can be misleading too, robbing you of
quality moments of life now for the promise of a quantity of life
after treatment.

I noticed through this whole process how easy it was for many of us to get hopeful, and of course it makes sense! We all wanted Peter to live. However, many of us didn't want to approach the most uncomfortable thought of all: what if Peter's treatment doesn't work and he dies sometime down the road, sooner rather than later? The choice was the comfort of the statistics versus the discomfort of Peter's possible and now more probable death.

The other side of this hammer of hope was Peter's tendency to keep a stiff upper lip. He stayed stoic, not wanting to burden family and friends with how it really was for him. Peter gamely put on the brave face. It was a noble yet ill-informed choice that our culture has so unkindly taught us to do. Don't be a burden! This stoicism hid the reality of how he was doing and was most problematic during his post-treatment stage.

It was difficult day by day for me. I could sense, as I sat with Peter, that all was not well in his body and that he was having a really hard go of it. But the brave face was on and he maintained that he "didn't have it as hard as everyone else on the fifteenth floor." After a few days of Peter's bravery, I felt compelled to have a little chat with him.

"Peter, sharing what is really going on for you is not a burden to me," I said directly. Peter looked a bit shocked and at the same time relieved.

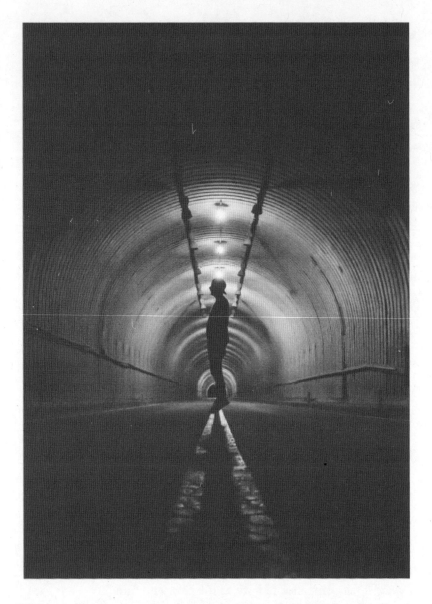

"I know you are having a hard time; it's obvious, Peter. Look at the chemo-cocktail you are drinking four times a day!" I continued. "The burden is being in this unreal place of you thinking I am thinking you are doing okay when we both know you are not." I sat quietly for a moment and let it sink in. "You have my permission to tell me exactly how you are doing and how you are feeling. It will not be a burden for me at all."

There was a silent pause.

"What is a burden is trying to figure out how you really are," I finished.

Peter's reply was short and sweet. "Okay, I'll do my best to be real with you." And he was, much to the relief of us both.

I saw how the hammer of hope and a stiff upper lip robs a family of important time to be together, just to sit and talk and say what needs to be said. This mallet is used to avoid the discomfort of saying good-bye just in case, to bypass all those potential lasts—our last text, our last phone call, our last hug. It is a tool designed to maintain our comfort level even though it is genuinely ineffective and robs all of us of deeper, more genuine human contact. In a way, misplaced bravery, coupled with a desire not to be a burden, disempowers our loved ones. Our behavior suggests they can't handle the truth, when in reality it is the truth that will set them free.

Different Points of View
Peter - posthumously

Peter came by his stoicism naturally; it was a kind of Garrett DNA thing. To be honest though, it is a pain in the ass. Here is an excerpt from an email Peter sent me in March 2013 that highlights and 'justifies' his brave-faced approach.

On 2013-03-22, at 6:53 AM, Peter Garrett wrote:

"As for informing people, I will do that at the time things turn even more serious (i.e. if my oncologist advises that things have deteriorated and he feels there is no other option than immediate chemo). I do this for a reason: No need to worry folks when there may be no need (i.e. the cancer may go into in to remission as a result of the alternative treatments)."

April

At this point, I am fully aware that the possibility of recovery is extremely small and so Peter's way of being in the world is not changing my ability to stay focused. What else can I do, anyway? Keep loving, keep loving, and keep loving, because that is what he would do for me. In many ways, this was the easiest stage for me. There was nothing else to do except live in the private and intimate world of suspending all thoughts, if possible, and focusing completely on responding to what was unfolding.

Stephen

I struggled with the hope thing a lot! I didn't want to be a downer and I wanted us all to be real too. It was quite a balance to find. I didn't want to take hope away from my family and friends, nor from Peter, and at the same time I didn't want to rob us all of precious time with him should things go south. I had seen it too often: Everyone gets involved in the fight for life. They lose the opportunity for graceful good-byes and quality time together now, thinking they will have a chance to do so in the future. Peter's bravado also got in the way as others in the family were kept at a brave-faced distance.

Why did Peter open up to me? Here is an excerpt from an earlier email that explains it.

On 2013-03-22, at 6:53 AM, Peter Garrett wrote:

> "That begs the question of why I have told you and no-one else in the family. I'm not entirely sure, except that you and I were hanging out shortly after I got back on this merry-go-round. Also, I believe that you can handle it better than anyone else in the family. It is nice to be able to talk with you, as you have such a great perspective on death and don't freak out about the possibility of my demise in the near future."

I realize now how important it is to be at peace with our own mortality. Who else can a dying person go to?

Yvonne

It's amazing how only a few pages of writing stirred up so many visceral reactions in me! I can't imagine how difficult it is seeing someone you love choose a path you feel is not the best choice, then stuffing your feelings down so you can be the best most supportive brother you can be! If all of the family and friends are cheering on the battle, who do you talk to about these unwelcome and raw feelings? Who do you turn to?

This is a critical piece of information that we don't seem to share openly. When we are sharing statistics, and how long people have lived after receiving treatment, quality of life is not part of the equation. Were they just alive or were they really living and loving their life? When did this stop being the most important part of the equation? I can tell you right now, if I had to choose between a shorter life with greater quality or a longer life of pain and misery, please, please support me and encourage me and love me in the decision to choose quality over quantity! Please do this for me, health care system and loved ones! Death is not failure, suffering is!

Stephen, thank you for having the courage to get to Peter, for letting him know that you didn't need him to be strong. You didn't need him to pretend everything was better than it was. We encourage that. Our society is scared to death of death. I've seen it at the bedside of the dying, and at funerals or visitations: "Oh, didn't she handle that so well? She was so composed!" Why do we feel that's the way we have to be? Why can't we be messy and vulnerable and grieve our hearts out? Let's be messy together!

Connie

The stiff upper lip is one embodied by most European-based cultures and I have seen it get in the way of a beautiful death time and time again. We see it in the news and in movies and it becomes who we are supposed to be. "He was strong; she was always so full of optimism and hope; he was the one who was dying but kept all the rest of us going."

I've seen this take place at the moment of death and far beyond. It robs us of saying what we need to say: the apologies, the sadness, the joy, the gratitude, sharing memories. When our loved one is gone, nearly everyone says, "I wish I'd said..."

I see people cry out in the hallway and then dry their tears and put on a smile as they enter the hospital room. What if Peter had allowed those tears to be cried in front of him? What if his family and friends had said,

"Hey, man, I don't want to be a downer, but there are some things I want to say, and then I promise we'll move on to something lighter."

I'm one to talk. I didn't cry for my mom when she died. I held it together for four weeks. Still, I had said all I needed to say. I hope that, between the stiff upper lips, Peter and his family managed to say what was needed.

Carrie

I knew Peter had only a short time left to live. What he decided to do was up to him, not me. I know he wanted more quantity of life. Personally, I was pushing for quality of life, and if it was me and my body, I would have chosen quality for sure, and that was not Peter's choice.

In thinking back, I wish we had spent a bit more time as a family having frank discussions about Peter's health care issues so we all could put our own cards on the table and as a family all be on the same page. Though each of us had a private chat with Peter, we didn't do it together, and as a result there was an elephant in the room when we sat together as a family. We all knew the end was near, yet Peter did his level best to protect us all from the reality of his dying. That was Peter.

That kinda' sums it up!

Marge

"Peter was always extremely determined. I remember how far he rode on his bike to get fireworks one year and then ran off to the park and put on his own show." He also never really showed any of us his pain," Mom reminisced. "To see him being so stoic was kind of natural. Peter always thought of others first, so of course he would behave this way."

"What was it like for you to see Peter lying in his hospital bed?" I asked, a bit tentatively.

"I didn't want Peter to see how distressed I was about his condition. I was so happy to see him and yet so sad about his really bad health predicament. It was hard to balance between what I really knew and felt and my desire not to burden him with my worries," Mom said softly. "I knew what the likely result was and in a way played coy so as not to worry or upset Peter."

CHAPTER FOUR

FIGHTING THE GOOD FIGHT AND THE BUSINESS OF CANCER

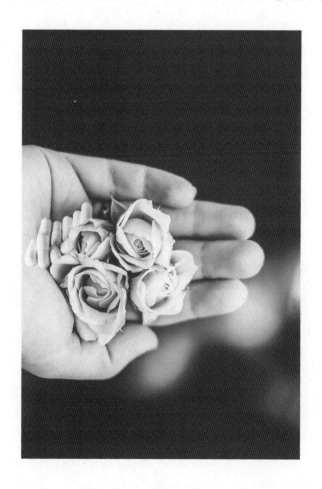

I was sitting in Peter's room on the second day of his chemo treatment. A nurse walked in to remove his empty bag and replace it with a new bag full of chemo juice. I asked, "By the way, how much does one of those bags cost?"

Her mater-of-fact response was shocking to me. "Between $30-80,000. This particular cocktail is about $50,000." It just rolled off her tongue like she was saying, "That will be $5.00 for your latte."

Wow!

Then add nursing costs, doctor's fees, other drugs, facility costs, food, maintenance, and administration. WTF! It's true we DO spend 50% of our annual healthcare budget on 5% of the people in the last ten months of their life. I was witnessing it!

The Business of Cancer

Here in Canada, we are very fortunate. We have an affordable healthcare system, well sort of, and provincial health insurance. We have access to treatments such as Peter's. However, it is important to know what treatments cost, along with all the other details, in order that we can make the best possible choice for our loved one's care.

Here are some examples of the enormity of the cancer business in North America.

> The splash page of the American Cancer Society starts
> off with Donate and Save Lives. The entire front page
> of their web site is donation driven. The society raised

$840 million in 2014. Of that, $276 million was spent on patient support, research expenses were $144 million, and administrative costs were $49 million, to mention a few budget lines. Fund raising costs were $177 million, or 21% of their annual budget.

The Canadian Cancer Society raised $198 million in 2014. Of that, $44 million was spent on research, $73 million on programs, $42 million in direct fund raising costs, $28 million in lottery fund raising costs, and $8 million in administration for a total of $78 million, or 40% of their budget costs.

Annual spending on cancer in North America was reported to be $124.6 billion in 2012.

Knowing all this, I asked Peter on one of his okay days if he would donate any money to any of the cancer societies. His answer was no.

"Why?" I asked curiously. Peter had been the recipient of extensive treatment over the past six years so I was a bit surprised.

"I am a dollar sign for them. Nothing has changed in fifty years regarding cancer treatments. We still operate, radiate, and provide chemotherapy, though we may be better at it with more efficient application of the same tools," Peter responded in a firm and thoughtful way. "We have not come close to winning the war against cancer, no matter how much money we have thrown at it."

When I was with Peter during the last five days of his life, we had some good chats. One was about his use of chemotherapy and radiation.

Looking back at the past six years of his life, he had some regrets. One was what he had done to his body.

We were alone in his palliative care room when he said, "I had to forgive myself for being so mean to my body. Looking back on it all, it feels like I tortured myself with toxic poison." Peter sat quietly for a moment. "I really don't think I should have done it. My body deserved much more respect than that."

We had a good cry together as we both felt Peter's deep personal regret.

Herein lies the dilemma: It's the good fight; it's noble and courageous. It's the right thing to do, to fight the devil we call cancer. Battle hard. Don't quit. We are making progress. We do save lives. We can win the battle against cancer.

The cancer societies' marketing campaigns and our fear of death are nasty bedfellows. Being frightened of death, we fight it at all costs. It is an easy sale, so to speak. However, it complicates the whole 'good' fight thing.

I have noticed over the years working with the dying that there exists an expectation that the one walking with cancer or a terminal illness will fight on at all cost and wrestle the monster of death to the ground. I noticed it with my brother Peter too. There is a subtle and sometimes not so subtle expectation that the one dying must fight for their life, that doing so is somehow more worthy than living the rest of your life as fully as you can without "having" to fight.

I watched a beautiful movie the other night, *Me, Earl, and a Dying Girl*. It was touching, raw, and thought provoking. In one scene, the teenaged girl fighting cancer decided she had had enough of treatments that were not working. She felt like shit physically, mentally, and emotionally, with no hope for a cure. She simply chose to stop the fight and live the life she had left.

When she made the announcement to her boyfriend, he lost it. He got angry with her for quitting, for giving up on college, life, and him. He yelled at her for making a choice he did not agree with. She asked him to leave if he could not support her in the choice she had made, and he did.

This raw and poignant scene speaks to exactly the point of this section of the book. Who gets to describe the good fight? Who has the final say? There seems to be a lot of people with tons of input from a multitude of perspectives, but all of it is only input. Some of it may be helpful and some of it may actually be a hindrance. At the end of the day who is it that gets to say fight or not, and how the fight will play out?

My brother was facing a difficult choice: Do I do another round of intense chemotherapy and then stem cell transplant? The whole system was involved: medical staff, family, co-workers, and friends. Now that is a lot of input! We all had different opinions, me especially. Yet at the end of the day, it was Peter's choice. Yes, we all got to say our piece, but then the important time came. Peter chose and we as his family needed to put our opinions aside and line up with my dear brother. We did and this is where the magic began.

Though I had a hard time watching Peter suffer, I was a big cheerleader for him. I simply took my upset to friends and family and shared with them my emotional reactions to what I was watching Peter going through. I kept myself healthy and served my brother on his chosen path. My emotional reactions about his choice would not have served him in any way. He already knew my perspective, so any further banging on the drum emotionally or otherwise would have been abusive. The entire family cheered Peter along and supported him in his choice. It was all about him, as it should be.

In his active dying, it was much the same. Once the 'good fight' was done and death was knocking on the door, Peter also had choices about how and with whom he would die, and he expressed his wishes clearly.

I guess that answers the question. Who has say about the 'good fight'?

The one dying does!

The costs my brother paid for fighting the good fight were not so much financial. His costs were much more emotional, mental, and physical. The most taxing, though, was the spiritual. He felt deeply in his soul that he had betrayed the sacredness of his body, that he was a bad tenant. Everything is right about wanting to live, to maintain your life and relationships. We do, however, need to be much more sober in our thinking and planning when it comes to facing both cancer and the slick, well-oiled cancer machine that seems to demand we battle on at all costs. After all, cancer is a business.

Different Points of View
Peter - posthumously

This sums it up for Peter, I believe: *Peter sat quietly for a moment and then continued, "I really don't think I should have done all the chemo and radiation. My body deserved much more respect than that."*

April

I asked Peter to forgive himself, to allow himself the space to make mistakes. That's hard when it's your life on the line! How can one transition gracefully and peacefully without self-forgiveness around choices made to survive? We all do what we think is best at the time. There are no right answers, as he was always quick to advise others. But at the eleventh hour, when this life is the thing that holds sway, it is so easy to forget what we know. Peter forgave himself. He let go of any judgment of the choices that he had made in his bid for survival.

Stephen

The fifteenth floor of Vancouver General Hospital is much like a war zone. I really didn't like it at all. It was the medical system on warp drive. Like a roller coaster, once you step into your seat and fasten your seat belt, it was full speed forward until the ride was over. Charts, nurses, doctors, administrators, numbers, drugs, machines, warnings, beeping, and buzzing; it was mind numbing and hard to find Peter underneath the cancer business. All this stuff seemed to come before Peter. Though I understood his choice—after all it was his life, not mine—I was disappointed for him and all of us.

I felt like he was being played by the system. I felt like a witness watching the movie of my brother's life. It seemed like cancer had positioned itself in front of and well before Peter.

Yvonne

There is a town called Lacrosse, Wisconsin, known as "The town where everyone talks about death." Apparently, most people have an end of life plan and they talk about death as the matter of fact that it is. Interestingly, they have the lowest health care cost at the end of life in the whole country. Why? Because they are not scared of death, and they don't make end-of-life decisions at end of life.

We are fortunate to have the health care system we have in Canada. But guess what? It's failing rapidly. The country cannot afford "free" health care at the rate we are spending the dollars. As the baby boomers age, we will not have the capacity to have everyone receive chemotherapy, or be on dialysis or in an intensive care unit to keep them alive. Then what? First come, first serve? A lottery? If we don't want it to come to that, we need to wake up and start diffusing the fear and denial of dying. We need to come to grips with the fact that we do not all die of old age!

Is chemotherapy big business? Is it about companies making a whole lot of money that would not be made if a cure were to be had? I won't say. All I know is this: if chemotherapy can save your life, and you can go on to live a life that you love, that's wonderful. If it is going to be an agonizing path just to keep you alive? I say we need to re-evaluate. As a nurse, part of a care team, I remember being wined and dined by a drug rep, encouraging our doctors to use their latest greatest chemo or anti-nausea medication. No expense was spared. The business of cancer does not impress me!

On to another subject. Peter's guilt about what he did to his body, how he felt he tortured himself, makes my heart ache. I know he was not alone in this feeling. I've watched more patients than I can count wither away to skin and bones, all in the name of not giving up. I have no doubt that they felt horrible about what their bodies were going through. Again, our society cheers on the fighter and sometimes it's like a badge of honour:

"I didn't give up. I didn't quit, no matter how much I was suffering!" I've heard it, I've felt it. I've seen patients in this state whispering to me that they wish they could just die, but their families weren't ready to let them go.

It hurts my heart. We can blame the system, the drug reps, the doctors, our loved ones, ourselves, or we can pause, reflect, and be a part of the change we want to see in the world of dying, death, and grief.

Connie

Making decisions before we have to make them is so important because we simply don't make our best decisions in the heat of the moment, when someone is hanging over us waiting for an answer. Doctors are taught and work in a culture of cure, and they operate through a filtered lens. Peter probably heard words like, "This is your only option," or, "You don't have another choice." Patients believe their doctors and they don't want to offend their doctors for justifiable reasons (I've had a few clients who were promptly 'fired' when they didn't like the options presented to them). Peter was making the best choices he could at the time. Regret comes later with the power of hindsight. I hope that he is now at peace with his decision to move forward with chemotherapy and that others are learning from his journey.

As for the business of cancer, I could get myself into some big trouble here. All disease care is run by big pharmaceuticals. I wish the Canadian pharmaceutical system was more like the US, where all of the side effects of the drugs have to be listed. It would make more patients pause and wonder if the cure or possible cure is worth the price. I believe in science, but the science is often ignored by those offering miracles.

Carrie

I think the health care system went to war on the cancer and left out the whole being of Peter. It was as if the system focused on cancer and somehow missed the humanness of him. I felt sad Peter as a whole wasn't being treated, only his disease was. It was as if he had become the disease and the rest of him had disappeared. I wondered who was caring for his emotional wellbeing and who was caring for his spirit.

Marge

"I found the nurses all very caring as they worked with Peter and handled their tasks gently and with care. They were doing their best to cure him," Marge said. "I found it interesting that Peter was mobile and able to visit his friends in other rooms. It felt like it was a caring place for him to be. I knew this is what Peter wanted and so the staff were giving it to him. It seemed to me the hands-on staff were on Peter's page and wanted to help him. I just wanted to be with Peter and support him in any way that worked for him."

CHAPTER FIVE

THE GOOD DAY
METER IS BROKEN

I have watched Peter through this whole journey, from the initial prognosis until his ultimate and graceful passing. I learned much by being his witness. One of the things I noticed as I went back over his six-year walk with cancer was that his internal meter seemed to become unreliable as time marched on and death neared.

It was his Good Day Meter.

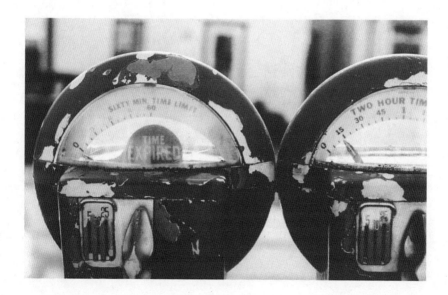

Here is an email to set up this chapter.

On 2013-03-22, at 6:53 AM, Peter Garrett wrote:

> *"Thanks for the messages, Stephen. I appreciate the concern and suggestions.*
>
> *Gurdev did call but we did not connect so I will call his cell today (Friday). He is correct: it is serious and it has been for a couple of years now. As you know, my concern about chemo/radiation is twofold:*
>
> 1. *they can both be carcinogenic in their right and*
>
> 2. *chemo is absolutely brutal on your immune system and independent studies show that repeated courses will kill you more effectively than cancer.*
>
> *Hence my desire to approach this using the best alternative treatments I can before subjecting myself to more chemo/radiation. I have not completely ruled them out as an option, **but I view them as a death sentence AND they will seriously impair my quality of life should this turn out to be my final act.**"*

Notice the date of the email; **2013-03-22, at 6:53 AM**

The damage to his Good Day Meter was demonstrated by his choice to undergo more rounds of chemotherapy in the fall of 2014 and chemotherapy combined with a stem cell transplant in May of 2015, only two years after he wrote this clear email. This is testimony to the impact impending death can have on the clarity of our thought process and our burning desire for even more quantity of life.

Earlier in his cancer days, a good day would be one with no sickness, some robust life energy, getting back to work, eating some good food, and enjoying friends. In other words, a day of remission looked pretty normal. The days, weeks, and years of treatment chipped away at Peter's Good Day Meter and blurred the scale of what good meant.

08-12-2015 Wed 11:22am

"Having a very low energy day. Otherwise okay."

08-14-2015 Fri 3:13pm

"Feeling a bit better today. Had a Skype chat with a friend. Went to town with April for breakfast and shopping. A great day given my challenges."

Over time, Peter's Good Day Meter became untrustworthy. The meaning of good changed according to where he was on his walk with cancer. He started to accept a mediocre day as a good day and then a poor day as a good day, and then one moment in a shit day as a good day.

An unreliable Good Day Meter is all part of the journey with cancer. This is why it is so important to have honest discussion with your life partner and loved ones early on. Have discussions about what values and quality of life you intend to have and what you will and will not tolerate. Importantly, to have them written down as a type of road map you and your family can follow, especially when things get messy.

The impact of extensive treatments affects both the body and the mind, and really does affect clarity of thought and tolerance. Peter used to refer often to his chemo brain, especially when I had just beaten him at cribbage! In some cases, it seemed to create selective hearing too! Here is an excerpt from another one of Peter's emails:

On May 6, 2015, at 6:30 AM, Peter Garrett wrote:

> *"After that, I have to stay in Vancouver for another month (again at the lodge) and have a 24/7 caregiver with me (thanks April and Carrie—you rock!) the entire time, while the specialists monitor my recovery. When that goes well, they set me free. I will return to our cute home in Wynndel to continue the recovery process. It will be at least 6 months before I can go back to work."*

Lots of things get fuzzy and unreal.

Now, I do understand the need for optimism, but it needs to be balanced with reality. This is exactly where and when family needs to be a rock for the one going through the process. This is why conversations about what we want and do not want from the medical system are so important. The advanced care directives that were completed in calm times now become our road map. Documents like this help all of us navigate the choppy waters that active dying brings.

It is not that we cannot change our minds and choose a different course of action; we just need to recognize where we once were and make well-reasoned choices, as opposed to the emotional and reactive choices many of us make at times like this. Often the family members themselves panic and make emotional choices for their loved one that were not a part of earlier agreed upon plans.

Sometimes, our own (the survivors) Good Day Meters have a sympathetic breakdown as we labor under the emotional, mental, and physical stress that active dying brings to all of us. We too can and often do settle for less quality. This is just another reason to have a plan that will remind us all of what our loved one truly wants. It acts as a road map as we drive down a newly explored highway.

Different Points of View
Peter - posthumously

Given it was Peter's own Good Day Meter that was broken, and we didn't talk about it before his passing, Peter has no comments to make at this time.

April

The broken Good Day Meter is otherwise known as hope. While appearing to gradually become less aware of what was good or poor or dismal, Peter began measuring his moments as a way to provide for his own quality of life. His spiritual goals were always to be aware and grateful for any light shining in an otherwise agonizing existence. Certain qualities over time became less important than they had been previously. The quality of feeling good was replaced by choosing to remain inspired by something; a way of maintaining a sense of himself throughout his journey.

Stephen

Looking back at it all, I find myself wishing we had done Peter's end of life planning more thoroughly—for all of our sakes. His stoicism and positivity deflected our attention away from what was truly necessary. I recognize, looking back, just how intricate and complex this whole end of life planning piece is. I missed some chances to support Peter more fully because we all weren't as clear around his end of life plans as we could have been. If I had a do over, I would have asked for the entire family to meet via Skype or conference call so we all could be more a part of the scene and stay on the same page. We needed to create some signposts by which we could be guided during challenging times.

Yvonne

Lowering the bar on quality—it's so easy to do when we are ill-prepared for grief, death, and dying. Sometimes we cannot accept that the person we love will not live as long as we want them to live. That is why the best time to plan and prepare for grief, death, and dying is when we are young and healthy. The next best time is now! I believe with all my heart that if we did this, if we planned our life and our end of life, and shared our values and beliefs with those we love, we would not lower the bar, and they wouldn't let us.

I have witnessed a good death, and I have witnessed a bad death. I can tell you that both are possible, but only if we have the courage to plan our lives and our deaths, and if we surrender to what is. We can grieve the life we wish was longer, our loved ones can grieve, but we do not have to suffer excessively.

Connie

Quality of life slips away like slow moving sand through an hourglass. Without a pre-made plan of when and how things will take place, there is no moment to say, "Here and now is where my quality of life is no longer adequate," or, "This is as crappy as I ever want to feel. Let's stop now." It's so important to say while you still have quality of life, "This is my line in the sand and I will not cross it." It is the adult's responsibility to put that in writing in an advanced directive so that it is clear to all involved, especially the ill adult, when that mark is reached. The adult can always change that line in the sand, but when they read what their former rational, healthy self said about the moment, it could cause a pause and re-evaluation.

Carrie

If Peter could do a few things on his laptop, have a little laugh, and perhaps eat a bit of food, this was a good day for him. I think his quality of life was tied into his pain being better medicated; the less the pain, the better the quality. I think that Peter really wanted his life to be okay so he acted as if it were, even though he was obviously dying and settling for a decreasing quality of life.

When you are that sick and on that much medication, it is easy to get out of whack regarding what a good day really is.

Marge

"I didn't really see him going through it all. Yet seeing your loved one for one more day IS a good day. This was what was important to him," Mom said. "It was his choice and if he got more days, then great. I didn't think it was swell and yet Peter did get more 'good' days with the love of his life."

CHAPTER SIX

SHIT, ROUND FOUR?
YES, ROUND FOUR.

On May 6, 2015, at 6:30 AM, Peter Garrett wrote:

Hey, everyone.

"I fly out of Whitehorse on Thursday, May 7, to go to Vancouver to start the next set of treatments. The first couple of weeks are all about the stem cell procedures and harvesting that goes until May 23. I will be staying primarily at the Cancer Care Lodge on W 10th—it is close to all of my many, many appointments.

After the 23rd, it is a waiting game to see when they can get me into the Vancouver General for the intense chemo. It requires an isolation room so that is why there is a delay of a couple of days to a couple of weeks. That process can go from 3 to 6 weeks, depending on how quickly I recover.

After that, I have to stay in Vancouver for another month (again at the lodge) and have a 24/7 caregiver with me the entire time, while the specialists monitor my recovery. When that goes well they set me free and I will return to our cute home in Wynndel to continue the recovery process. It will be at least 6 months before I can go back to work.

Best time for visitors would be before the chemo starts or when I am back in Wynndel well on my path to restoring my immune system. I am thinking September onwards but need to check with the doctors on this as there are sooo many things I am not allowed to do in recovery, i.e. no Sushi!! No gardening (bacteria in the soil), etc. etc. I need to find out when I am cleared for visitors.

I will have both my laptop and cell phone with me so feel free to stay in touch, BUT don't take it personally if I do not reply quickly—I may be in the midst of a rough patch.

Admittedly, I am a tad nervous about it all, but also excited to get going with this so that I can move on with the next phase of my life (figuring out what I want to be when I grow up).

Hope you are all doing well. Take care.

Love,
Dad/Peter/your favorite nickname for me..."

When I picked Peter up at the Vancouver International Airport, the man I saw walking towards me was not the Peter I remember, but an old man laboring his way painfully to the baggage claim carrousel. I noticed it each time I was with him. Our walks to and from the Cancer Care Cottage were painful and slow. Watching him getting up and down a six-inch curb was hard to witness. Getting into and out of a chair was always labored. Though Peter was only sixty-one, he appeared to be closer to one hundred and one. It was hard to watch and likely even harder for Peter to be in a body that was becoming less and less able.

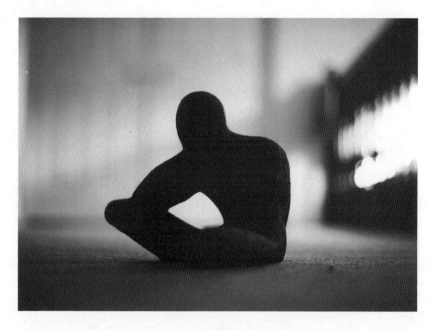

It felt like time was precious so I made strong demands of family to get out and be with Peter, likely for the last time. Thank goodness they all responded with a resounding yes. On May 20, I picked my mom and sister Carrie up at the airport and drove them to my place in Maple Ridge. My sister Sue had arrived three days earlier and was staying with Peter at the Cancer Cottage. April arrived under her own steam and was staying with friends in Richmond, a little closer to the Vancouver General Hospital than Maple Ridge was. The Garrett clan, the remaining five from the original seven, was together again.

We had a wonderful family barbeque on May 21. We laughed, told stories, teased, and had a grand old time. Mom was Mom and continued to mother her sixty-something children, and we kids, as always, rebelled. Dinner finished, conversations completed, and dishes done, we whisked Peter off to the Vancouver General Hospital's Bone Marrow Transplant Ward as he readied himself for his intensive chemo and stem cell transplant treatments. None of us realized then that it was our last Garrett family gathering with Peter. One or two of us may have silently thought it, but it was never spoken aloud. Though everyone was optimistic, there was an underlying and unspoken feeling that this could be Peter's final hurrah.

On May 22, 2016, Peter took up temporary residence on the fifteenth floor, the Bone Marrow Transplant Ward of Vancouver General Hospital (VGH).

Now for a bit of Garrett family 'inside' information. My brother loved coffee and knew the inner workings of hospitals pretty well. Their coffee was nasty! In order to enjoy the smaller things of life, he brought his own coffee maker to the hospital and installed it right beside his bed. Great coffee was now guaranteed and very close at hand!

As I walked into the cavernous lobby of the VGH, I was reminded of my time with a dear friend Daniel, who had faced a similar prognosis as my brother and had graced the hallways of the fifteenth floor a year earlier. Daniel had died on that very floor after an agonizing final six months of fighting cancer. I tried to set my experience with Daniel aside and remain open to a different outcome for Peter.

I stepped off the elevator onto the fifteenth floor and found my way to Peter's room. I immediately noticed the biohazard sign on his door and the biohazard waste can placed just inside his room. Peter was resting comfortably on his bed drinking a recently brewed cup of coffee with his new friend Paul from a few rooms down the hall. Paul liked good coffee too.

We three sat and chatted. The conversation ultimately focused on the biohazard warnings plastered on Peter's door and the all over the garbage can. Cytotoxic Waste, the signs read. Though they were ominous, our collective senses of humor ultimately ruled the day, and the Cytotoxic Café was born. A sign saying so soon hung just above the coffee maker, much to the amusement of most everyone who entered the room, aside from Mom, who thought we were being a bit irreverent. She did manage a smile all the same though.

Peter's chemo treatment was still a few weeks away, so the Cytotoxic Café had time to flourish—and it did! His room was the site of many great coffee shop chats amongst fellow patients, and from time to time, staff, friends, and family.

The first month of Peter's time at Vancouver General Hospital and the Cancer Care Cottage were spent stabilizing his body, doing all sorts of scans and tests, and compiling masses of health data from which the cancer care team could plot out a course of action. Then sometime during the first week of June, the team and Peter took the plunge: four bags of chemo a day for six days!

I remember walking into Peter's room and seeing him plugged into the system of tubes and bags and beeping machines that contained all manner of drugs and fluids designed to kill the cancer with minimal collateral damage to the rest of his body—at least that was the plan. He looked like shit and his color was that kind of yellowish sick grey that people get when death is hanging around.

As I stepped through the curtains and past the biohazard can, I said, "Hey Chemosabe, how is it going?"

My brother immediately responded, "Not so good today, Taunto."

Mom, sitting in a chair by Peter's bedside, chided me for being cruel at such a time and Peter immediately rode to my defense. "Mom, it's okay. I feel better when I laugh."

The rest of the time was a blur of treatments, charts, numbers, and prayers. Family members gradually headed home and on July 22, 2015, Peter and April set out in their car to return home to Wynndel, BC.

Different Points of View
Peter - posthumously

"Wait for the results was all I could do, and waiting was really tough work," he said days after his return home.

April

Love Peter and wait for the result was all there was for me to do. I knew the end was near.

Stephen

This was a rough time for all of us, watching Peter go through yet another round of intense chemotherapy. It was hard to watch him suffer through all the nasty side effects, the headaches, the sickness, the diarrhea, and the body pain. I was horrified at the drugs, not just the chemo, but also all the other drugs they used to manage all the side effects chemo brought on.

It was also hard to see Peter be swamped by all of it and in a way smothered by what was going on around and because of his illness. It was like Peter took a seat in the back of the bus and cancer was riding shotgun. Often nurses would come in to his room and get right to work barely even noticing on whom they were working.

I made it a daily habit to always ask the nurse for her name and then introduce her to those of us in the room. I wanted there to be some humanness in the room that was otherwise flooded by technology. I felt like I was losing Peter to the health care system that he was somehow being swallowed up and eclipsed by.

Yvonne

Peter was so incredibly fortunate to be a part of this family—wife, sons, brother, sisters, mother, friends—who were willing and able to put their lives on hold to be there for him. They put their own angst, discomfort, and pain aside to show up for this man that they all loved. What a gift. That last Garrett clan gathering? Priceless.

I think of the many people I've watched over the years, battling cancer and endless treatments alone. So very alone. I can't imagine what kept them coming back. I believe that in many cases, it was the fear of death, seeing it as the worst possible outcome. I wonder, is it really worse than suffering in isolation and loneliness?

On a lighter note, I love the Cytotoxic Café, irreverent or not. Never ever lose your sense of humour. It's one of our greatest gifts.

Connie

I will only address this as a nurse because there were obviously so many dynamics at play during this difficult period. I am so glad that Stephen introduced the staff to Peter's humanness, because the lack of it in a hospital drives me quite nuts. There are rules and rationale for everything: gowns, gloves, and masks (this one is obvious in Peter's case); why you can't bring in pillows or blankets from home (they could get lost; they are germ ridden); why you can't wear your own clothes (ease of examination and nursing care); why some flowers aren't allowed (other patients' allergies). Pretty soon there's nothing left of the person and only the patient is left behind. I'm so glad to hear about the coffee machine but if someone in maintenance had found out about it, it would have likely been taken away (could cause a fire). Just saying.

Carrie

I was there with my mom and my sister Sue when Peter was going to have his stem cells harvested for transplant. We stayed with my brother Stephen, his wife Sonora, and his in-laws Dan and Diane, who were so wonderful throughout everything. It was a family reunion of sorts, and a wonderful time for us all to share and remember, even though I knew it might be the last time we all saw Peter. I was there for five days, then had to return to Ontario for work.

Once Peter's stem cells were reintroduced, he was to stay in the cancer center in Vancouver in isolation for six weeks as the cells were reintroduced to his body. Peter was on a limited diet, and isolated so as not to cause any risk of harmful toxins or viruses to get into his body and kill the new cells. I was elated and sad all at the same time, as I knew the risks and possible outcomes of this treatment.

I was amazed at how positive, strong willed, and real Peter was with everything he was enduring. I wanted with all of my being for Peter to be cancer free once and for all. I hoped and prayed for his journey with cancer to end on a positive note. The stem cell transplant seemed to be moving along well and so Peter was able to go home to Wynndel with April to finish his recovery.

I was asked to go and stay with Peter and April for a couple of weeks while he was recovering, so April could work and not have to be going 24/7. I gladly accepted and flew out to Wynndel in July. It was the most awesome time for me to reconnect with Peter and April. I learned so much from Peter about his cancer journey, the choices he made and why, and how he felt through it all. I was honored to be a part of his journey, and to be able to help in any way I could. I was able to offer a few Reiki sessions to both Peter and April, if they wanted. I enjoyed every moment of each day with them while I could. I had to return to Ontario knowing it would only be a short while before I headed back to BC to see my BB again—this time for his last journey with cancer.

Marge

"Mom, what were you thinking and feeling watching your son go through these medical treatments?" I asked.

"I was hoping for the best for Peter. I didn't want to give up hope. It was hard to see him in pain and looking so ill," Mom replied. "It's really hard for me as a mom to watch a child of mine so sick and looking like death. Staying hopeful for Peter and at the same time knowing there is a good chance he will die was hard for me to balance."

CHAPTER SEVEN

BACK AT HOME WAITING FOR "NORMAL"

Peter was back home in Creston and the waiting game was in full swing. Waiting for results, waiting for normal, waiting to feel better, waiting to start living again. Waiting, and waiting, and waiting.

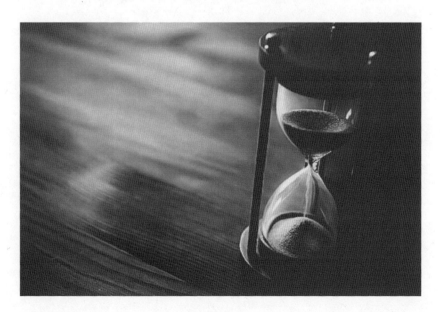

Out of my love for him, I thought it might be a good time to begin writing this book. Typing on a keyboard might not be too draining, and the exercise of writing might give him something to do to feel somewhat productive. It might be cathartic and helpful emotionally too. I sent a text to Peter.

07-21-2015 Tue 6:50pm

> *"I have begun writing Chemosabe and Taunto Riding Sidesaddle with Cancer. Will send you the draft chapters and perhaps, energy willing, you can begin to join me in the writing of it."*

My hope was that having Peter write some would help him get back into his life with a bit of a purpose. Perhaps it would be an emotional lift too. Well, not to be for the moment at any rate. Here is his reply:

07-21-2015 Tue 8:59pm

> *"I will have to get back to you. This recovery thing is harder than I expected. Exhausted, in a lot of pain still, and emotionally drained. I know things will improve but I am feeling overwhelmed and useless at the moment. Do not need a pep talk. I understand these things quite well in my noggin. Just need to be patient and keep putting one foot in front of the other, and give my body the rest it needs...*
>
> *Ttyl"*

I found myself thinking that this is the way it could go for the rest of Peter's life. A few days later:

07-25-2015 Sat 5:38pm

"Peter how r u?"

07-26-2015 Sun 7:57am

"Same. Lot of pain; can't sleep. Not a good dynamic. Ah, well. No one said it would be easy...

How's byu?"

It was clear to both of us that Peter was in a deep health crisis and had little energy for anything else but rest. The book, if we were ever to write it together, would come much later.

We were waiting for normal, or results, or anything to suggest a break from the pain and sleeplessness. No such luck; the pain and lack of sleep went on and on. A week later:

08-04-2015 Tue 5:59pm Peter wrote;

"Have not heard from any of the Vancouver doctors since I left. My Whitehorse doctor (the amazing Sally) let me know recently that my LDH levels (among other things an indicator of cancer growth) have increased significantly over the past month. So, I have a call in to the Vancouver doctors to find out whether this is normal at this stage or whether I should be a bit concerned."

08-05-2015 Wed 8:10pm Stephen wrote:

"Thanks for the update. Sending you love. Anything I
can do for you from here?"

I was the only family member, aside from April his wife, that Peter felt inclined to be raw and real with. He needed an outlet without having to alarm the entire family and I was it. His email said it all, three weeks after leaving Vancouver General Hospital and still no contact. Here is some of what he was dealing with:

- Challenges dealing with the medical system

- Long distance emails with distressing news

- Uncertainty and no more normal

- A fleeting hope that normal will return

- No communication forth coming from the medical system

The great unknown was looming in the foreground—again! Though Peter was in the medical system, he seemed to be all alone in it and in some odd way unseen by many of those who claimed to be serving him.

Here is a text he sent to me that demonstrates this weird sense of not being seen by the people within the medical system paid to serve him.

08-13-2015 Thur 4:56pm Peter wrote:

"Spoke to the Cranbrook Hospital this morning and
they say they never got the request for my scan. So, I
called the Creston Hospital and they are going to resend

*it. I will double check tomorrow. Otherwise just tired
from the pain and not sleeping enough."*

Four days later, I sent a short text to Peter.

08-17-2015 Mon 2:46pm Stephen wrote;

"Hey Peter... what's new? Xo"

Peter's reply.

08-17-2015 Mon 5:10pm Peter wrote;

*"Hospital finally got the scan request so hopefully I
will get in over the next few days. Still too much pain
and not enough sleep. Really affects everything. Do not
like it."*

08-23-2015 Sun 10:27am Stephen wrote:

"Any news on the scans yet?"

08-23-2015 Sun 4:48pm Peter wrote:

*"No. But I spoke with my oncologist Dr. Villa on Friday
and he is going to talk to the hospital in Cranbrook."*

This lasted from July 21 to August 23, 2016. It was over a month of
waiting to get back to normal and this is all Peter had to show for it!
There was nothing but uncertainty and little or no support from the
medical system to help him know and understand what was real in his
body. All the indicators were pointing to bad news and yet no one was
able to help confirm our worst fears.

These fears were not often spoken of, by the way. Most of my family members, including Peter, were clinging to the hope that the stem cell transplant would work and that these tough times were "normal."

Watching Peter go through these challenges in a weakened state was a real wake up call for me. I began to realize just how much we all needed to take personal control of our case as we attempt to move through the system successfully. If no one is advocating for us, it is like the blind leading the blind. If I want a good result, I need to be my own champion or have a loved one champion for me—perhaps hiring a patient advocate.

Now we were into the second month of recovery after stem cell transplant treatment. All Peter's efforts to get his 'normal' back are going sideways again. He has serious and difficult pain to manage, especially in his left leg. His blood counts are showing negative signs too, including rapidly rising LDH levels that could be signaling the resurgence of cancer. He went from the Creston Hospital emergency room to Cranbrook Hospital for scans, with a potential trip back to Vancouver General Hospital for more intensive exploration.

If cancer returned, the medical system's response would likely be palliative care, as the fifteenth floor Bone Marrow Transplant Ward was the last stop for allopathic treatment for Peter. Pain management and quality of life would be the guiding forces in his care if the reports and tests are negative.

I am the only family member aside from April to know what's really up for Peter. My sister Carrie has a feeling something is wrong, but everyone else is in the dark and hoping for good results. Peter will let them all know once he has some concrete information to share as he doesn't want to alarm anyone unnecessarily, but his gut body feel is the cancer has returned. His spirit is crushed again!

Here is the content of an email Peter sent to me while I was in Singapore teaching.

On Aug 29, 2015, at 8:56 AM, Peter Garrett wrote:

"Glad things are going well in the city-state.

Had blood work and x-ray done Tuesday and the CT scan Wednesday. All due to having an amazing doctor in the Creston ER take me seriously when I went in Tuesday morning (at April's insistence). Even better, he has agreed to adopt me as an orphan patient so I won't have to go to ER except for tests.

Waiting for the official phone call with all the results but he indicated my platelets and hemoglobin are very low. Given they are both blood related I am blaming the blood thinners. He was inclined to agree but didn't want to overstep the thrombosis doctor on this.

He also put me on a new pain med (Gaba Pentin) that is working really well and has the added benefit of making you drowsy so I have actually had three nights of good sleep. As a result, I am feeling better mentally and physically.

We have a friend visiting today and tomorrow from Cranbrook, which is fun (she and April are currently beachcombing for rocks and driftwood—I would just slow them down so stayed home for that). We may have more friends arriving right after that.

So, life is good.

All the best and much love, Peter"

Reading between the lines, it doesn't look good. Days later, I received this email from Peter as I was on my way home to Vancouver:

On Sep 2, 2015, at 2:28 AM, Peter Garrett wrote:

"Yo, bro!

No idea where you are but perhaps en route. Let me know when you are back.

Test results are in and not good. Mainstream medicine is washing its hands of me as far as treatment goes and shifting completely to palliative. Will be calling Mom et al to let them know verbally so please do NOT post anything to your FB or other media 'til I have done that. Thanks.

Take care.

I love you, Stephen,
Peter"

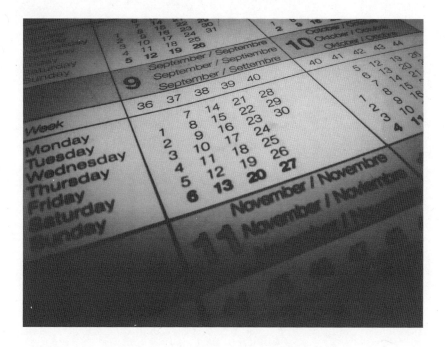

My intuition and concern had just been made real by one simple sentence, and I am sure Peter had the same kind of visceral reaction only much deeper level than mine. After all, it was his life that had just been put into question.

The death sentence had been delivered. Peter was given two weeks to two months to live.

Different Points of View
Peter - posthumously

With profound reluctance, Peter accepted the death sentence and oddly a state of grace became noticeable. The fight was over.

April

Now what I have known all along shall come to pass. Again, some physical arrangements, nursing considerations, and healthcare provider paperwork have to happen. Stay focused to get that stuff done. Stay present for Peter. Don't take anyone's crap, and ask for what I need. Very basic, to the point functioning for me. The bubble feels like it's getting larger, less encompassing, but more expansive, a moving away from the physical and into the spiritual realm. It is time now for the important work of letting go so Peter can transition peacefully and consciously.

Stephen

Feelings of relief, anger, and sadness cycled through me. I was angry at Peter for being so stoic. I was relieved that soon the battle would be over. I was sad that I would be saying good-bye to Peter forever. I was angry the treatment didn't work for him. I was feeling sad for April and my family especially for Mom, and in a way I was relieved for all of us. Soon the struggle would be done.

I planned my trip to Creston Hospital for the final days with Peter.

Yvonne

The waiting game is one of the most excruciating parts of this journey: the unknown, the lack of communication, the feeling that the cancer is back every time you feel a twinge. This is another large gap in the system of compassionate care. We need a better checking in routine when patients are no longer receiving treatment and are awaiting results. You should never feel abandoned.

Another one of the greatest difficulties is feeling useless and needing care, as Peter experienced more than anyone really knows, I would guess. I wonder if planning for and being prepared for that overwhelming sense of uselessness would make a difference.

Hearing how much Peter endured, how his spirit was crushed over and over again, is so difficult. Sadly, it is a common story, but one that chips away at the hearts and souls of us all. It makes for an end of life story that saddens everyone. We all have much to learn from these journeys—patients, families, friends, and medical staff included.

Connie

I work with a palliative support foundation and what Peter experienced with the oncologists is a sad day-to-day occurrence. In the best of worlds, Peter, his wife, and family would have been referred to palliative care long before his final treatments. Palliative care is not the same as hospice care, though they are often on the same trajectory. All should see palliative care as learning to live life at its fullest until the day you die. It supports patients and families to learn how to cope, to grieve, and to move forward, even on bad days. Really, Peter was discharged into home hospice and the process and the result are different. One is living well with terminal illness and the other is dying well. I would love to see the medical system use palliative support much earlier so that there is a continuum of care. It sounds like what Peter and his family needed.

Carrie

I was home for only a short time when I asked Peter if he had any word from the oncologist regarding his cancer. You see, while I was out helping

Peter and April in Wynndel, Peter was having so much pain in his hip that it was hard for him to do his usual daily routine, which was to heal and enjoy the nature that surrounded him. Peter became exhausted so quickly that I was very worried. He was so stubborn and never complained about the pain, but his face and body language showed it all. I would cry in bed at night, and pray for an end to his pain. Peter was strong, but the cancer was stronger. Before I left, I reminded Peter to call his oncologist to book an appointment to get his pain level checked and have those tests run that he wanted done.

Back to the question I asked Peter: had he heard from his oncologist regarding his test results? Peter's answer was heart wrenching. The cancer was spreading very rapidly, and was very aggressive. He had between two weeks and two months to live.

I cried and yelled at the universe, and yet deep within my heart and soul I knew it was best and kindest for Peter. He was in great pain and suffering. His body was being taken over by a cruel and nasty invader! It was eating him alive. Peter was so thin and pale, and wasn't eating much at all, if anything. It was with great honor and deep sadness that I returned to Wynndel for my last visit with my BB.

Marge

"I had a feeling that this would be the end for Peter when I left him at Vancouver General Hospital. I was so glad we did have some quality time with him and that BBQ at your house, Stevie, was such a special time for us all," Mother said. "It was hard for us all too. I am glad Susie came to visit me. I was happy not to be alone when that call would come in telling me Peter had just died. That is really something a mother doesn't want or expect to hear, especially all alone."

CHAPTER EIGHT

THE BEGINNING
OF THE END.

The full court press was on and cancer was in total control. Our worst fear was now made concrete. God bless our doctors, but they tend to over-estimate these sorts of things by about 50%, I guess in a way trying to soften the blow. I did some quick math and concluded I had best get my ass out to Creston so I could spend a few last days with Peter. I was guessing he had two to three weeks at best.

Carrie flew out from the east, I drove in from the west, Mom stayed put in Ottawa, and sister Sue headed to Ottawa from Nova Scotia. We didn't want any of our family alone at this time. It was important to us all to be supported by loved ones as we all faced Peter's dying together.

I arrived at the Creston Hospital around 6:00pm Monday evening. Carrie was in transit. I found my way down the hall to the Butterfly Room, the hospice room for palliative patients. I had been in many such rooms, but this time it was different: *it was my brother dying*. I paused outside the room. I could hear April and her sister Amy talking with Peter and

I didn't want to go in. It seemed almost too real, surreal if you will, as if it was a movie scene from someone else's life.

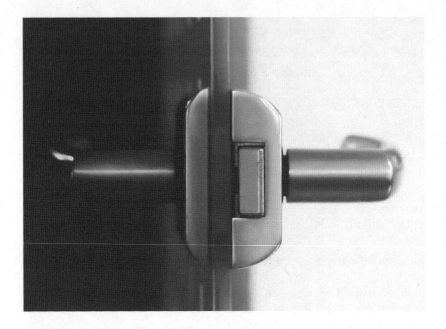

I took several deep breaths, opened my heart, and poked my head into room 18 at the Creston Hospital. April and her sister Amy were tending to Peter, massaging the aching parts of his war-torn body. He looked old, haggard, and grey. His thin body was propped up by pillows on one of those hospital beds that contort into many shapes and angles. His meager offering of hair was much like baby hair and white-gray in color. His checks were hollow, his body fragile and barely mobile. Each movement looked painful. His dinner was left untouched. He had tubes in his arms for painkillers and hydration.

He looked like shit, God bless him. Though he was alive, it was clear death was close at hand. He was present though and able to talk. He did so with huge effort, and mostly to keep his visitors at ease.

We said our hellos and cried a bit at the rawness of the end that was coming ever closer. The girls and I caught up. Peter was able to get up with assistance and he chipped in his two cents as we chatted. His contributions were concise and infrequent, a sign of his retreating life energy.

It was late evening now and by this time Amy had picked up Carrie from the airport in Cranbrook and was driving back to the Creston Hospital. Carrie arrived and she joined right in. Having spent two weeks with Peter in August when he first returned home, she knew the ropes and her way around the hospital, Creston, and Peter's home. It was good to see her again, even given the circumstances.

We spent the night at the hospital and stayed most of the next day, evening, and into the early morning, then finally went home for a short nap. It was dark when we arrived at Peter's place for my first visit there. A long and narrow driveway led us down into the acre and a half retreat-like site. The home was rustic and lovely, much as April and Peter had described it, as was the guest cottage I was to sleep in.

In the midst of their living room sat Peter's home hospital setup, hospital bed, night table, and all that sort of medical stuff. It felt strange to see at first, an odd setup for a living room, yet given Peter's health needs, it made total sense. It was much as I thought a home death setting would look. The bed was placed strategically in front of a large living room window, looking out over the beautiful Salmo-Creston valley, as I would discover in the early morning light. There was a fabric room divider to provide privacy, I assume when he was napping and guests were over.

The guest cottage was comfy and I fell asleep quickly, exhausted physically by my long drive to Creston and emotionally by the events of the past days.

We returned early and not so bright the next morning with coffees in hand. I was surprised by how much Peter had changed in just a few hours. He was still able to chat and move about a bit, just not as easily as he had done only a day earlier. Peter's mother-in-law, Pat, was there, as were Amy and April. Carrie and I said hi, and we all hugged and visited with Peter.

By early afternoon, talking was over, meals were a thing of the past, fluids were done, and his body was continuing to shut down. It seemed like he was collapsing in on himself. His color was even paler. His breathing, though steady, was labored, and body movements were now performed with assistance aside from the occasional arm or hand gesture. His lungs were struggling as fluids started to build up, demanding even more drugs to limit the congestion and ease the pain. He had trouble clearing his lungs and gurgled a fair bit. We sat together, chatted a little, but mostly just sat quietly and loved each other.

Carrie and I went for a late lunch a few hours later, and returned energized and refreshed after a lovely all-day breakfast. We returned just in time as arrangements were being made for Michael, Peter's son, to fly out from Winnipeg. My credit card came in handy. Darren, his other son, was already organized and would be arriving early in the morning by car.

We said good-bye to April's mom, who was heading home to Alaska, and rejoined Peter for a late afternoon visit. Conversations were shorter than Monday's, as Peter was noticeably more tired. He wasn't eating and couldn't stomach the Ensure drinks. He was having trouble swallowing. After chatting with April and Peter, we decided to stop the hospital food from being delivered. It was time to begin letting go of life even more.

We took over the hospital room and had a chat with the nursing staff. We wanted to minimize all the coming and going so we could settle the room down for Peter's active dying. We intended to create a sacred and calm space. April, being an LPN herself, knew just what to do. Working with the nursing staff, we were able to create a bit of a sanctuary that felt a whole lot better than the prior medical busyness. Interestingly, the nurses seemed relieved and pleased in a way. They felt the love, care, and commitment we all had for Peter's graceful passage, and were happy to give us the space we wanted and that he deserved.

As the day wore on, Peter began to drift away. Though gamely present, it was clear death was coming much sooner than any of us had imagined. April sensed his growing fatigue and we chatted about how we could organize all the visiting in a way that would give family a chance to be with Peter and give him the rest and quiet he wanted and needed to prepare for his death.

Darren, one of Peter's sons, and his partner arrived late Tuesday evening, more likely early Wednesday morning. The Winnipeg kids were arriving just in time. The room was full of people so Carrie and I decided to call it a day and headed back to Peter's house for a much-needed sleep, though short it would be.

Early the next morning, we returned to Peter's bedside. His eyes were clear and he was still there, but not much else was functioning. Peter now communicated mostly with his eyes, along with some grunts and groans and some facial expressions that April was skilled at interpreting into English for us. His body temperature was on the hot side so a cold wet towel adorned his head. His body was more and more lifeless. There was no movement in his lower limbs, rare hand gestures, and occasional facial gestures were all he could muster. Cheeks sunken, feet puffy, color almost non-existent, head and eyes, ever more still.

We took shifts sitting with him. The room became still and Peter slipped in and out of consciousness. Often his eyes were closed. Sometimes, rarely, they were open. His breath became a little more erratic as each hour passed. I could hear the rattle in his lungs. He, his essence, was in his body, but only barely. He lay on the hospital bed leaning to his right, motionless.

There was nothing to do but love him and wait.

Death felt just around the corner.

In moments of quiet, sitting with Peter, I thought about the sweet times we had all shared over the past days. I remember seeing all of our hands placed on Peter, on his arms, hands, legs, and feet, as we did our best to comfort him with loving healing touch.

I recalled seeing April kiss the top of his head tenderly as she gave him permission to die. It brought tears of sweetness and sadness to my eyes.

I recalled a scene with Carrie and her hands on Peter's feet, Amy with her hands on his chest and heart, offering the gift of gentle, loving reiki.

I remember Carrie and me sitting in the hall outside Peter's room looking out over the Salmo–Creston Valley crying as we had a chat with Mom. We talked with sister Sue, who had arrived to keep Mom company at her apartment in Carleton Place. I recall how sad it all felt and yet how very much love was present, surrounding Peter and our family at this important time.

I remember Darren and Michael sitting at their father's bedside crying quietly with their dad, who was able only to respond with a sparkle in his eyes.

I remembered fondly my drives with sister Carrie to and from April and Peter's home in Wynndel and the hospital. Carrie navigated while I drove and it was a time for quiet sharing.

We had waves of deep sadness and feelings of profound love; sweet and sad at the same time.

More family arrived on Wednesday. Peter's son Michael and his gal would be flying in from Winnipeg a little later in the evening. By 9:00pm, the room was full of people, emotions, conversations, and visiting, which began taking a toll on Peter as he did his noble best to greet family and well-wishers with at least a sparkle in his eyes. Carrie and I decide to head back to Peter's place and give the boys some privacy with their dad. We noticed his life energy was waning and the sheer number of people in his room was clearly wearing him out.

Back home for a short Wednesday night sleep, we returned to the Butterfly Room Thursday morning at 8:00 am with coffee in hand for April. Stepping into the room, I saw an even more diminished Peter. He was totally still, eyes now deeply cloudy and eerily vacant, with no sparkle at all. His breath was slow, unpredictable, shallow, and labored. I felt as if I was looking at a cadaver. His body was barely alive. Peter, his essence, was nowhere to be seen or felt in his body.

April, ever present with him, knew better than most that today was the day. The room had taken on a sacred and quiet tone and visits were kept short in honor of Peter's wishes to die privately with only his wife present, if possible.

My last visit with Peter was around 11:00 am, just he and I. His face was sunken and unshaven, and he sported scruffy grey-white stubble.

His breath was barely audible, body absolutely motionless, and an eerie vacant look in his eyes, almost haunting in fact. I held his face in my hands. He was a little cool to the touch. Looking into his eyes, searching for him, I saw only a body. It seemed as if 'Peter' had already left. I kissed his forehead, said I love you, and left him as sunken and motionless as he was when I walked into his room earlier in the morning.

"Until next time, dear brother," I said with tears running down my cheeks.

I walked away from Peter for the last time. Turning and looking back over my right shoulder, I saw the hollow shell of a once vibrant and alive man. I smiled and cried at the same time. I knew him once. In that instant, I understood the quotation, "Parting is such sweet sorrow." Shakespeare knew of what he wrote!

With all the good work the family had done, Peter was on his way, held for days with loving, passionate care and fondness. Now it was only a matter of hours for his body to let go and catch up with Peter's earlier departure. I said my good-byes to one and all. It was time for me to go; there was nothing else to do.

The drive home was still, silent, and reverent as I spent those hours privately saying good-bye to Peter, heart-to-heart and soul-to-soul.

Moments after arriving home, I received this text from April:

09-17-2015 Thur 8:45pm April wrote:

"He's gone"

An entire life of sixty-one years ended with such a simple phrase. It is how Peter wanted it, alone with only wife and sister Carrie by his side. Simple, graceful; no more, no less.

I wept with both sadness and joy: sad because he was gone and joy because I had known him. I shared the news with Sonora, my wife, and my in-laws.

I went to bed and fell asleep relieved that Peter and all of us were now free from his painful struggle for life, and yet missing him deeply.

Different Points of View

April

I spent the last five days of Peter's life with him in his bed or in the chair beside the bed. The bubble was now very large and filled with light. Right up until the last twenty minutes of his life, we spent five hours wrapped in a cocoon of light and love. "Remember who you are and that you are divine. You are not alone. I will be fine, I will miss you like crazy, I will always love you, and you will always love me. This is not the end, but a new beginning. You get to go on before me, don't get too far ahead, eh?" No words, just feelings and that golden white light. When I saw his face, I knew he was free. He had a smile on his face and his expression was the same as when he found something particularly delightful, his eyes crinkled up. I kissed his eyes shut and we anointed him with oil. We sang him a journeying song. I collapsed on the couch and stared at him on the bed. I felt a rush of energy move through my feet, all the way up through my body and out the top of my head, like a wave of ecstasy. It was his good-bye, and only as he would say it—with the passionate joy of a truly beautiful man. I have been blessed! I have been blessed!

Stephen

I spent Peter's last days with him. It was a touching and intimate time and it was a very uncomfortable time too! The sacredness of the dying process, the family supporting Peter, and the friends sending well wishes was remarkable and loving. My family felt the support of our friends around the world. It was awe-inspiring and soothing to our aching hearts.

The uncomfortable piece for me was witnessing my brother's active dying—not so much from a mental, emotional, or spiritual level, but mostly from a physical perspective. My body recognized Peter' body—DNA. You see, we came from the same two donors. It felt as if I was watching myself die! Though I had been around a lot of death and dead bodies over the years, including seeing my father Lloyd's and my sister Jody's dead bodies, I didn't witness their dying process. My body didn't get to experience looking at its own death. The rawness of it, the reality of it was very uncomfortable physically and yet the experience was profound and in an odd way freeing. I felt like my body somehow faced its own ultimate death, shook it off, and was now free to live.

Odd though it may sound, my brother Peter's dying and death somehow freed me up to live even more fully, and more passionately.

Yvonne

Why do doctors tend to error on the side of optimism instead of realism? Is it to give the family hope? Is it to stay positive? I'm sorry but I think it is mostly selfish and a way of not having to face the painful message they should be delivering. Why not be as forthcoming and honest as possible? Why not error on the side of pessimism? Then, if by some miracle, a cure is to be had, celebrate! If you have said your goodbyes, planned and prepared for end of life, all the better. You will have shared some beautiful moments and you'll be that much more prepared when death does indeed arrive.

Stephen, when going to see his brother Peter for the last time, took a deep breath and opened his heart. To see someone you love "collapsing in on himself," knowing that it is at last time to let go, is beautiful and painful. The best thing you can do? Just show up and love. That's all that's left to do.

This was such a long hard journey for everyone. I'm so glad this wonderful family had the insight to want to create a sacred and calm space (it would have been even more wonderful if that had been created for them). He was enveloped in love, kindness, and tenderness. Everyone placed their hands on Peter to comfort him, and that moment even makes me smile. I can feel the love for this man.

Peter finally left that tired, diseased, broken body. A beautiful family was left to grieve the man they loved so much, and to find their new normal.

Connie

I truly hope that Stephen realizes what a massive gift he gave his brother and the family. By knowing what a good death can be, he brought that to his brother's death and any negative (guilt, anger) grief were likely substantially diminished from what many families experience. Nothing can protect us from the impact of seeing the ravages of a dying body no matter how many deaths we've witnessed and a death from cancer is incredibly cruel.

To Carrie, I hope to one day meet you. I was at the bedside of both my parents as they died but I would have given anything to have known how you helped Peter pass and that he did it through you. What a gift.

When I was a maternity nurse (almost thirty years ago) doctors were the directors of birth. They came in for the last few minutes to deliver the baby but it was the nurses who toiled with the mothers for endless hours. At that time, midwifery was just making its massive resurgence. Now, few doctors are involved with birthing and I feel that it's just as well. I would like to see that happen at the end of life too. It is not a place for doctors who have not done their own death work. Only seasoned, compassionate doctors who realize that death is not an enemy to be conquered should be teaching the new physicians on when hope and optimism are no longer appropriate. It robs patients and families of time to grieve and say goodbye.

Well done, Garrett family. It was a gruelling journey but one you will take with you for the rest of your lives. You will help others who are living with dying, families and friends, and others, like me, who have been asked to come along on your journey.

Carrie

April had already started the hard task of letting family and friends know that Peter was now dying, and had merely days to live. April's sister Amy was there to support and help April and Peter in any way she could. She was a wonderful blessing, as was all of the family and friends that showed up. We went to the hospital daily. Peter was admitted to the palliative room, as his complex care needs needed attending to. It was wonderful to share in Peter's last journey on this earth with family and friends around. We laughed, cried, and got angry too.

I was utterly amazed at the strength, compassion, and love with which April cared for Peter every moment of every day. April was there from the start of Peter's cancer journey, right until the end. I am in awe of her great spirit and strength through it all.

On the evening of September 17, 2015, April called Amy and me and asked for us to come to the hospital so she could have a rest. I was on deck with my BB for one last time. I told April and Amy I would be there to help Peter let go and leave this earth to be free of all his pain and suffering once and for all.

Amy took April out of the room to the car where she could cry, scream, laugh, and just let go.

I was so honored and blessed to be able to be there for Peter. I took his hand in mine and told him I was there, how much I loved him, and how honored I was that he wanted me there for his last journey and breath of life. This was Peter's time to take his big leap of faith and continue his journey on the other side.

He gave his grunt, "Ummmph," which was him being stubborn. I reminded him that he had said he would take that leap of faith when it was time. Once again I got his stubborn grunt. "Ummmph!" I said, "We'll count to three, you'll take that last wonderful breath in, then on the exhale, you'll let go."

He sure took a breath and a leap, and I thought he was finally at peace, but he came right back! Stubborn Irishman! I kid you not, Peter came back! I damn near jumped out of my skin. I even told him that if he took that wonderful leap of faith, I would do my happy dance for him. I guess he wasn't ready to see me dance! Peter must have found it funny. I asked him if he got a glimpse of where he was going, and he "Ummmphed" quite emphatically, which I understood as a yes!

My response was, "Now that you know where you are going, can we try it again?" Once again, Peter "Ummmphed" and gave what looked like a grin, along with a sigh. He was ready now. "So on the count of three, BB, you will breathe in then take that awesome leap of faith on the breath out, okay? One, two, three." I heard my amazing BB take that last breath. I felt his wonderful energy pass around my body as he finally took that leap of faith to leave this world for a wonderful pain-free new journey on the other side.

And so, as promised, I did my happy dance for my BB's final journey home.

I love you and miss you with all of my heart and soul, BB! I have never been more proud of you than I was when we spent our last moments alone together on your final journey home.

Love you forever and a day, Carrie.

Marge

"I was so glad that you and Carrie were in Creston with April and that April's mom and sister were there too!" Marge said quietly. "It is not good to be alone at times like this. I am glad that you and Carrie kept Susie and me up to date. I know those telephone calls we hard on us all and sad too, but they were important to keep us all together on the same page with Pete."

Mom sat quietly for a while. So did I.

"It was a sad time for us all. We once were a family of seven and soon we would be a family of four. I can't help but wonder who will be around next year," Mom said.

"And to think I am still here." She sounded surprised.

CHAPTER NINE

END OF LIFE PREPARATIONS AND CREMATION

On Tuesday, two days before Peter's death, April and I decided it was time to go and make the funeral arrangements so all would be in order well in advance of our needing their services. I wanted to support April in this way, and didn't want her to face it alone.

I'm so glad we did it together.

I think there is only one funeral home in Creston and it was just down the street, two blocks from the hospital. I remember walking in the front door of G.F. Oliver Funeral Chapel and flashing back to my year and a half stint as a cremationist in a funeral home in Vancouver. It felt oddly similar. It had the same kind of setup, familiar feeling, and the arrangement room looked like most of them do professional, neat, and orderly with a dish of candies on the table.

The automatic doorbell chimed. Guy Roy, a soft-spoken gentleman, greeted us in the lobby and took us to the arrangement room. He left for a moment, giving April and me time to settle into the space. It was a small room with all the usual trappings. Behind the curtain was an offering of all manner of caskets and urns—not for us though.

When Guy returned and sat down, he asked, "How can I help you today?" It was an odd question, I thought, given we were in a funeral home. I told April I would be the spokesperson for us, so I began.

"My brother Peter is up in the hospital nearing the end of his life. April, his wife, and I would like to arrange for his cremation." I spoke in a clear and measured voice.

I surprised myself. Though I had sat through many funeral arrangements in the past, never had I been involved in such a direct and personal way. I was making arrangements for my brother's cremation! April and I had discussed all the necessary details prior to meeting with Guy, so I confidently moved forward with the conversation.

"Guy, we want a basic cremation: cardboard casket and no frills. There will be no service or viewing and I would like April to be at the crematorium if she so decides," I said, taking total charge of the situation.

I didn't want April—or me for that matter—to be soft-sold or up-sold or marketed to in any way. We knew exactly what we wanted and what we didn't want. No fancy caskets that would send Peter out in style and empty his bank account. Money up in flames? No thank you. There would be no services in the chapel, as we had our own celebrations of life planned.

Guy looked a little disappointed, and yet he felt our clarity and certainty and prepared the contract exactly as we wanted. It was $3,500 for a basic cremation. They were the only funeral home/crematorium in town, but in Vancouver a basic cremation was around $1,200. April was not at all surprised by the price and quickly signed the contract.

In a stroke of a pen, it was done. Peter's arrangements were made.

Guy asked us to let the nursing team know they should call him once Peter's death was pronounced. I took his card and agreed to do just that. We stood and shook hands, said our farewells, and we were on our way in just over thirty minutes.

Heading back to Peter's room in the hospital, I stopped by the nursing station and let the nurses know to call G.F. Oliver upon Peter's death. They nodded kindly and made a note on his chart.

G.F. Oliver Funeral Chapel handled my brother's cremation with grace and dignity. I am thankful for their support and service, as is April.

Different Points of View
Peter - posthumously

Peter was clear that he wanted a no frills cremation. Being frugal, he wanted to ensure the minimum costs with the most of his money going to his surviving family members. He had made sure April was clear on his wishes.

April

We both knew what Peter wanted for him after his death. Keep it simple. No big deal. Cremation. Family celebrations to follow when it was right for us all.

Stephen

I was well prepared to support April in dealing with the local funeral home. I had spent a couple of years in the funeral business and knew how arrangement meetings were handled and what to expect from the funeral director. April and Peter's clarity around what they wanted was a great foundation to negotiate from. I kept it short and to the point, leaving no room for up selling or marketing.

Emotionally, it was just weird. I was happy to support April in this way, very sad to be making these arrangements for Peter, and angry that it was so expensive. It also had a surreal feel to it. Peter was dying and death was very close!

Yvonne

I can imagine what it feels like to walk into the funeral home to discuss arrangements, knowing that the death of your loved one awaits. Thank goodness Stephen was able to be there with April so she did not have to have that talk on her own. I'm grateful to hear that Peter's cremation was handled with grace and dignity ($3500 for no frills—really?). Let's look at a different scenario, my wish for the world:

Peter and April find each other, fall in love, and marry. They make their life together and they plan their end of life, discuss what is important to each of them, make decisions about organ donation (if they haven't already), and make certain that their families are aware of their decisions. They include the boys in these conversations. All is in order.

At the end of Peter's life, which has arrived long before anticipated, long before anyone is ready, everything is in place. All that is left to do is to let him go, and to begin to grieve the man they loved so much.

The day April and Peter went to the funeral home to make the final arrangements looked very different. Everything was already done. Instead they took that time to sit by the river or hike up a hill, or whatever they needed to do to care for themselves and each other, knowing their long journey through grief was about to take another turn, the final letting go.

Carrie

I was totally on board with Peter's ideas to go out with no frills. Yeah Peter!

Marge

"I was happy you were there to support April with these sorts of hard things to do alone. I have handled a few for your father and my sister and it was trying," Mom said with a sigh. "And of course, with your experience in the funeral home, you would have known the ropes. Glad it was you there helping April out."

CHAPTER TEN

BUSTING THE MYTHS ASSOCIATED WITH GRIEF

When you spend enough time around dying, death, and grief, you notice something: We each do it differently.

Each dying process I have had the honor of witnessing has been totally different. Each death is its very own. Each journey with grief is uniquely personal.

Yes, there are some common signposts that you can rely on, stages you can count on, but they don't follow any particular order, nor do they show up in the same way for different people. There is no tried and true formula.

It depends on a multiple of factors ranging from age, gender, culture, and the relationship with the deceased, to mention just a few. These variables and the uniqueness of each person's personal belief system, upbringing, and life experience demands we practice the art of dying, death, and grief support.

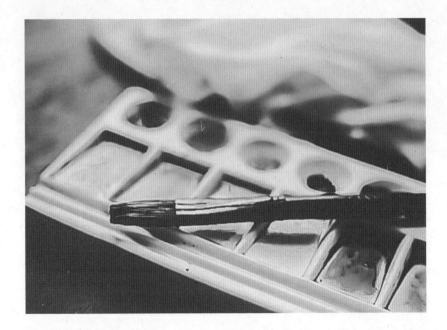

People often look for the one map of grief, so we make them up. Yes, the charts help, but only to notice the different facets or tendencies. There is no one map or one way. The two maps below highlight what I am saying here. The one on the left displays what most of us hope for, because it would be easier to handle and much cleaner to process. The one on the right demonstrates what it is really like: messy.

All of us—men, women, children, and elders—grieve, we just do it differently. We each have our own unique squiggly road map of our grief touching on each of the stages for sure just in our own way, our own personal order, and in our own good time.

The opportunity for those of us drawn to work in this remarkable field of dying, death, grief, and loss is to become a great artist with a large and diverse toolbox of experience, training, and attentiveness. There are many paint brushes, and lots of colors, so we can choose the right brush with the right color combination for the person (canvass) in front of us.

Paying attention and not knowing is a great approach to take. Let the individual in front of you inform your selection.

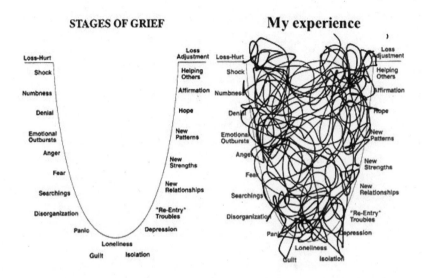

I have also noticed a disturbing tendency in both the one dying and those grieving. Many of us believe our grief is a burden to those around us. It is another myth that clouds this much-misunderstood field of dying, death, and grief. It is linked to our poor relationship with death based on the outdated model of the grim reaper—another urban death myth.

The emotions of grief are a gift, not a burden. From personal experience, I know this to be true. Grief is simply an outward expression of the love we had and still have for the deceased. It is love redressed, love in a different costume, love expressed in a different emotion. We are taught to share all the lighter emotions and to hide or suppress the darker ones; those, we are led to believe, are a burden.

This is another opportunity for those of us drawn to this work to reframe dying, death, and grief so people can see there is a more fulfilling and satisfying way to die and to grieve. Other cultures do; all we need to do is a bit of research and a lot of practicing of new dying and grief habits! It all starts with you the reader deciding to change your relationship with dying, death, and grief to turn towards the grief instead of turning away from it.

Here are some of the books I have read that really helped:

1. **Permission to Mourn** by Tom Zuba

2. **Seeking Jordan** by Matthew McKay

3. **Turning Toward the Mystery** by Stephen Levine

4. **Preparing to Die** by Andrew Holecek

5. **I Found a Dead Bird** by Jan Thornhill (for children)

6. **The Toltec Art of Life and Death** by Don Miguel Ruiz

7. **The Tibetan Book of Living and Dying** by Sogyal Rinpoche

8. **Dying** by John Hinton

9. **At The Edge of Life** by Richard L. Morgan

10. **The Afterlife of Billy Fingers** by Annie Kagan

11. **I'll Shave My Head Too** by Steve Dolling

12. **Die Wise** by Stephen Jenkinson

Some movies I have watched that were supportive were:

1. **Departures** - https://en.wikipedia.org/wiki/Departures_(2008_film)

2. **Tuesdays With Morrie** - https://www.amazon.ca/Tuesdays-Morrie-Greatest-Lesson.../dp/076790592X

3. **Me, Earl and a Dying Girl** - https://www.imdb.com/title/tt2582496/

4. **Stepmom** - https://www.imdb.com/title/tt0120686/

CHAPTER ELEVEN

THE GIFTS DEATH
LEAVES BEHIND

"How Did Death Become My Greatest Teacher?" I asked myself one day not so long ago.

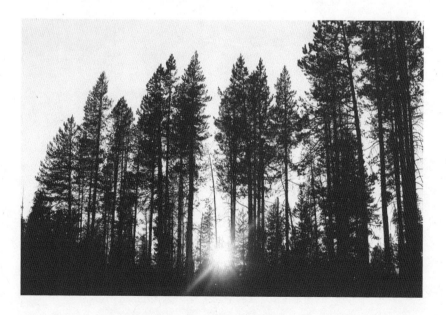

When I look at the image we adopted for death here in North America, I am surprised that my own picture of death, my own relationship with it, is totally different. I hold death as a wise grandfather, an almost exact opposite to the more commonly held vision of a grim reaper. I consider death a successful birth of sorts, while the medical system considers it a failure. How the heck did I come to this image of death?

My first experience with death that I can recall was with my Grandpa Joe. The details are a bit sketchy, but it didn't go well. I recall he fell at home, broke his hip, went to the hospital, and never came out. The funeral was weird too. The adults didn't want to answer my simple 'kid' questions: "Why is Grandpa's skin cold?" "Why is he wearing a suit and tie?" "Why does he have makeup on?" "What is he doing in a box?"

It was awkward and no answers were forthcoming. I felt like a nuisance and the adults all looked stunned. It was a bit like I was an unwanted child at an adult affaire. I was sent outside to play with the other children.

That was it. Done. Never spoken about again.

I guess I pushed all that stuff down and out of my mind. I don't recall any other deaths clearly. Uncle Eric passed away, as did his wife Kaye. She died first, I think, and my memories are not at all clear. There was a car accident and a few of my hockey buddies were killed. It was weird that little was said in the locker room. It was like they just stopped showing up to play. I remember a few pets, for example Sam our beagle and Ginnie our poodle, being put down and all of a sudden not at home any more, with nothing much being said. This just seemed to be the way it was; someone died and life went on as normal.

I must have filed it all neatly away in my mind and body never to see the light of day again, at least until my dear sister Jody died on May the 5,

1988. The whole ball of dying, death, and grief I had neatly tied up and hidden away began to come undone.

Jody's passing was significant for me. It was the first family death I had to face as an adult. I had to tell my parents that their daughter had died. I was a pallbearer. I had to face Jody's extended family and friends, a funeral home, a church service, and a burial in the cemetery in St. Catherines, Ontario. I had to adult up. I remember holding it all together, keeping a stiff upper lip, and thinking how crazy that was. She is my sister, she is dead, and I am lowering her body into the ground. I felt like bawling my eyes out, and yet held it all back.

After all was said and done, I simply couldn't hold it all together. I went to a therapist to get some professional help with my grief. Death was still bad and wrong and needed to be fought at all costs. Oh, I bargained with my therapist, I negotiated with God, I offered the Universe all my money. I offered God my Ping golf clubs, which included a one-iron I was told only God could hit. I offered my therapist my life if only Jody could live. All my bargaining was to no avail. There was no deal to be had. Jody was dead and I needed to deal with that reality. I did, and in the midst of my grieving, I stumbled on the most remarkable gift: my own wonderful life that I could live my own way.

Jody died and I woke up out of my North American slumber! A year later, I quit my Bay Street job, moved west, and started a career in social services.

This was my first real experience of discovering a gift left in the shadows of a death! I miss Jody to this day and yet I am grateful for her passing. Her death woke me up to the reality of my life. Perhaps death wasn't quite the enemy I thought it was.

Next went Dad.

Ah, the old fella had been sick for a while. A long life of drinking, hard work, and hard play took its toll on Lloyd's body. He simply started to break down. He died in the hospital after the family and he agreed to unplug him from life prolonging machines. It was February 8, 2004. Lloyd was 78.

I will always remember what Dad said to me during our last conversation.

"Son, keeping me alive like this is not loving kindness.

Unplug me.

If I live, I live.

If I die, I die.

I want to go out on my terms."

Lloyd's funeral felt different from Grandpa Joe's. Yes, there was a viewing, as there was for Grandpa. There was a service, as with Jody. Family, friends, and church were involved too. People said eulogies, and there was food at home afterwards. Actually, it was very much the same as Grandpa's funeral, now that I think about it.

Why did it feel different then?

Oh, I was different!

Yes, my own relationship with death had been fundamentally altered by Jody's passing. My willingness to look more closely at dying and death had enabled me to accept death as a natural and fundamental facet of life. It may not have been complete yet, but progress toward a new relationship with death was well underway.

The gift Dad's passing left behind for me was taking full and personal responsibility for my life.

I became a hospice volunteer in 1992 and have been volunteering since then. I was also a cremationist in 2012/13 for a funeral home. I immersed myself in the field of death as a volunteer and as a professional. I wrote a book entitled *When Death Speaks*. All of this was my way of giving to my community and befriending death. I have seen a lot of it, even before the death of my dear late brother Peter on September 17, 2015.

I was indeed well prepared, though not quite ready for his passing.

His death was truly graceful. His six-year battle with cancer not so much, but the final week of his life was indeed special and sacred. His fight to live, his dying, and his death have been some of my greatest teachers, and have opened me up even more to the powerful tool of being present to dying and death. I became even more aware of death's power to educate each one of us about life—if, that is, we are open to the lessons death has to teach us.

Peter's dying and ultimate death was uncomfortable for me. The discomfort I experienced was a reflection of the potential gift that was to be left behind once he passed. I have learned the greater the discomfort the greater the gift.

I had seen my sister Jody's body, and my late father Lloyd's corpse, both laid out in caskets; however, Peter's active dying was the first family member's dying and death I had witnessed. It was uncomfortable because I was watching my own death, if you will. My body felt Peter's dying differently because he and I are of the same DNA! While watching his passing, it became clear to my spirit, my mind, and my body that there was no way out of life but death! In a way, I became death clear.

I sat with both Peter and my discomfort. All I could do was love him, breath, and allow his dying to bring us closer in love and to inform me more about how to live life. I simply sat and opened myself to what was unfolding as Peter moved ever closer to his last breath.

Peter's dying and death left behind the gift of a question: "Did you live as passionately, lovingly, kindly, and fully as you could today?"

Death has changed for me over the years. It is no longer the grim reaper it started out to be. It had morphed into an inspirational teacher. It didn't happen overnight, and there was no quick fix. It just took time and an ongoing intention to embrace death, to get to know it, to learn to live in harmony with it, and to live with the certainty of my own death.

A Gift for You, the Reader
The Three G's for Healthy Grieving

Grief is sticky, a bit like those double-sided tape rollers used to remove lint from sweaters. Unresolved grief tends to act like a magnet and attract your more recent grief to stick around. This goes on under the radar and below our consciousness. It is not that we want to hang on to our grief, more that we have forgotten how to fully clear it out of our system. We accumulate pieces of grief from different types of death and it all gets stuck together under the surface.

I notice a low-grade unhappiness in people that I believe stems from our inability to grieve well and completely. Sometimes some of us aren't able to recognize we are experiencing grief at all. It is also a result of the lack of meaningful and practical rituals in our busy urban lives.

Below is a list of mini deaths or losses that most often are not recognized as worthy of grieving, and yet grief, our natural human response to loss, is ever present, whether we acknowledge it or not.

Loss of employment - Loss of relationship -Loss of ability or capacity

Loss of childhood -Loss of adulthood - Loss of money

Loss of a limb - Loss of youth - Loss of energy

Loss of appetite – Loss of a pet

Loss of personal freedom

Loss of identity

Or

Change

The **first step** to becoming personally grief resilient is to acknowledge that change, such as the examples above, does lead to a natural grief response.

The **second step** is to create a special place in your home that you can go to grieve the losses you experience in your everyday life.

The **third step** could be to create a special space in your garden that you could use as 'cemetery' for the losses to be buried.

Here is an example.

I lost my job and though I was angry initially, I realized I was actually sad. I was grieving the loss of my pay cheque and a part of my identity. I allowed myself to feel the loss and wrote of my experience in my journal. I created a paper object that represented both the cheque and the job. I burnt it as a mini cremation and then I buried the ashes in my garden.

As simple as this may seem, it worked for me. I created a ritual that allowed me to acknowledge the loss, to grieve it, and to bury it so I would not carry it around with me and add to it with other losses. In other words, I put my grief garbage out for recycling!

As I buried the ashes, I did so with a feeling of gratitude, as best as I could muster. I gave thanks for the pay cheques, for the opportunity to work with my work mates, and for my newfound freedom (this piece was tough initially!).

I also looked at what I had done in my estimation to bring about the firing, along with what I think I could have done to avoid it. Guilt.

In handling the **three G's**—grief, guilt, and gratitude—I was able to move forward in my life without the anchor of the loss holding me back.

Acknowledge the **grief,**
Check for any subtle **guilt,**
and
Process all of it with **gratitude**.

The Final Chapter

Peter Eric Garrett
Celebration of Life
August 7, 2016 – Whitehorse, Yukon

April set up a Facebook page called 'Peter Garrett Celebration of Life' as a place we could all go to remember him. Here are some of the comments placed there by friends of Peter.

"Peter's love and care changed a life half way across the world. He sponsored Kechelet for four years through Little Footprints Big Steps (founded and led by Peter's young friend, Morgan), giving him the opportunity to experience hope, dignity, health, and an education. Kechelet has a photo of Peter on his wedding day near his bunk bed and a mango tree has been planted in the Safehouse garden in his honor."

—Karen Wienberg

"Peter made me feel special every day. I miss him a lot. Thank you, April, for so generously sharing him with us. Linda's picture captures Peter perfectly. I will look through my photos as well."

—Bev Land

"This was taken one Saturday morning around 9am last August, outside of Burnt Toast in Whitehorse. Peter and I were heading in for breakfast and a visit. This is how I saw Peter and how I will always think of him. So proud to be Irish, and we all know how much he loved to debate an issue. I miss him every day. What I am most grateful for today is that I have April in my life."

—Linda Steinbach

"Blessed remembering my favorite Irishman! Anyone remember him dressing up for St. Patrick's Day?! Those emerald colored shoes?"

—April Garrett

My tickets are booked, it's July 13, 2016, and in less than a month I'll be in Whitehorse, Yukon, for the celebration of Peter's life. The formal date is August 7, 2016. Mom and Carrie have purchased their flights, as has April, but sister Sue can't make it.

I am excited to meet Peter's friends and colleagues, folks I heard about a little yet never met. People that know him in a way I do not. I thought I would feel more sadness and may still once I have landed in Whitehorse, yet in this moment I am filled with curiosity and an interesting feeling of joy, sharing Peter and memories of him with folks who loved him as I did.

Yesterday, I was hanging out in my garage, pouring through a trunk full of family photos and memorabilia, looking for photos of Peter that I could take with me to Whitehorse. It was a fun thing to do. It was sad because Peter was not with me while doing it and fun in that I got to review my own life through the wonderful collection of stuff my mother had so carefully sorted and kept. I have some great pictures to share with family and friends. They are part of a scrapbook I am taking with me.

This scrapbook will be a place for family and friends to remember Peter in a written way, and with their permission will help form the final chapter of this book dedicated to his life. With some help from my publisher, you will find their hand written entries on the closing pages.

It is July 26, 2016, today. The trip to Whitehorse is days away. Time to get packed.

August 4, 2016. Vancouver International Airport Boarding Gate 20. WestJet Flight 503 bound for Whitehorse, Yukon. I am a tad nervous, actually, thinking about the hundred or so people that will be attending Peter's celebration of life. I'm looking forward to seeing Whitehorse, I've never been there, though through Peter's stories I feel like I know it somehow. I would like to go to his old office and see where he worked, whom he worked with, and what it was like for him to live and work there.

April, Peter's wife, is already in Whitehorse helping to get things organized for the big day. Mom and Carrie are on their way tomorrow. It's true that births, marriages, and celebrations of life bring us together as families and as communities. It's the power of love in action.

Laura's house. Wow, I am in Whitehorse, Peter's town!

I drove by where he worked, through his town, on streets he used to walk. I saw the hospital where the great Doctor Sally works and where he received some of his chemo treatments. It was cool and weird at the same time.

Dinner tonight is at Laura's home, and who knows what Friday will bring. She is such a generous host and did really love Peter. We had fun chatting about him and about life in the Yukon. We spoke about the maintenance man in the building where Peter worked and how he was so thankful for Peter's help from time to time with legal things.

Friday and Saturday were a bit of a blur, with Mom and Carrie arriving and meeting many friends of Peter. We had dinner at Don and Jan's family friends of April on Friday; touring the city of Whitehorse on Saturday; visiting the hall for Peter's celebration; and yes, another family dinner on Saturday evening. It was all done in the love of community for dear Peter.

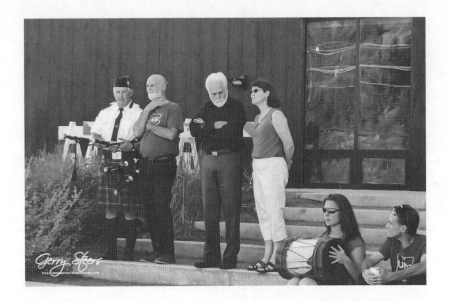

Sunday morning arrived and all the planning for Peter's life celebration was falling nicely into place. A bunch of us were at the hall down by the river setting up for the day. April was handling the altar. I was taking care of the memory table, and a group of folks were in the kitchen preparing for the potluck. It seemed that all of a sudden, people were beginning to show up.

Marge and Carrie arrived at about 1:30 pm and that opened the flood-gates. By 2:15, the place was full and the celebration began. Andy McLeod played us in with his bagpipes. A short movie of Peter's life was followed by numerous stories about him from those in attendance and also many from others sent by both mail and email. April's good-bye love song to Peter was followed by a beautiful outdoor ritual that sent Peter off on the waters of the Yukon River, under the watchful eye of a bald eagle that showed up just as April was sprinkling Peter's ashes into the river. It was the first and only bald eagle we were to see all weekend.

Andy piped Amazing Grace and we all, in our own way, let Peter go. The group was held in the loving sunshine of a warm Yukon summer's day.

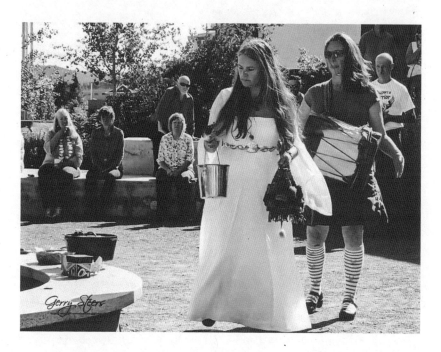

We slowly made our way back into the hall for the potluck dinner and many more stories of Peter. A sound track of his favorite music played in the background. The memory scrapbook was a popular lingering spot, as was the food table! Warm hugs were the order of the day, as were heartfelt conversations. I met Sam, the shy maintenance man, and exchanged telephone numbers so we could text hockey insults back and forth—a habit he and Peter once enjoyed. Thank goodness my Montreal Canadians are on top of the league this year!

Slowly and gracefully, the hall emptied and we all made our way home.

The day was done.

Peter was let go and free to soar.

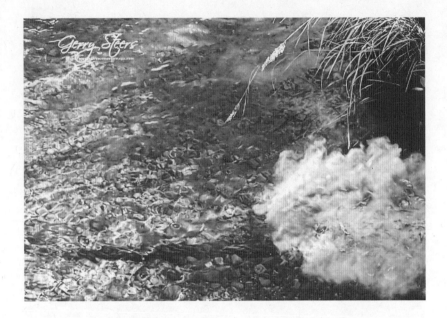

Until next time, my dear brother Peter, until next time.

It takes a village to let go well.

The following pages contain many of the love notes people left behind and some closing posts on Peter's Celebration of Life Facebook page.

"Remembering Peter today from afar. I'm so happy we got to know this amazing man who inspired us to be better and more loving humans. XOXO"

—Tracey Nobes

"Hello to all attending the Celebration of Life for Peter. Wish I could have been there in person. I will check Facebook and YouTube later in case any of you post videos from the event. My best to everyone and thinking today about our good friend Peter. I know he is watching over all of us and sending positive energy."

—Art Hay

On September the 17, 2016, one year after Peter's death, the Facebook page died too!

Here are some of the original notes in the Memory Scrapbook from the August 7, 2016, Celebration of Peter Eric Garrett's Life.

 Gmail
TSquare Architect <tsquarearch@gmail.co

Fwd: Kevin's Message
1 message

Shari Borgford <shari.borgford@gmail.com>   Sat, Aug 6, 2016 at 12:20
To: "T-Square Architecture Ltd." <tsquarearch@gmail.com>

second one....

Subject: Kevin's Message
To: "shari.borgford@gmail.com" <shari.borgford@gmail.com>

"Hello, and my regrets for not being among you all on this day of celebration in honor of Peter. In my absence, I have put a few thoughts to paper and offer it to share.

There is some great irony as I write this reflection on Peter. Firstly, last two conversations we had were on the topic of being in far foreign lands, actively pursuing one's desire to live out one's dreams and travelling around. I am writing this from an empty beach, on a far-away island in Thailand, and secondly, it was Peter who contributed to get me thinking about leaving my job, of which it was 3 years ago today, I left the government after a long career.

Peter was a great human being. We only shared coffee twice, which was such a long time ago now, but I remember it was in the Broken Spoon cafe, now long gone. The first time, he asked me out, to chat about lessons in how take leave without pay for extended periods and how I went about finding one's purpose. Peter apparently had also wanted to get away and do something different overseas, that aimed to bring some good to others in need. Unfortunately, our 30 minutes went by way too fast and it back to work we returned. I clearly remember that he picked up the bill and him telling me, that he admired my global sojourns to foreign lands and my wanting to help people, because I actually went out and did it, rather than just talk or complain. The second time out for a coffee, probably years laters, was me asking him out, in order to learn some things about the pros and cons about the quitting the federal government, then coming back and the financial penalty, as Peter was well versed in that topic. Again, our 30 min coffee went by too fast, but he offered me his overall experience and his circumstances. As we prepared to leave, I will always remember him looking at me seriously and saying, "you know Rumsey, you can walk away before you turn 50 year old, think about it, get the f*** out, you don't belong here in government land, the world needs you"....three years ago today, I left my job.

I didn't know Peter that well, we were just fellow colleagues working in two different departments. first time I saw Peter he had a long pony tail, somebody then told me he was a lawyer, and I remember thinking how cool is that, a bureaucrat lawyer with a pony-tail. However, what stands out most about Peter was his super personality and how each and every time he passed by my office, he would acknowledge me in a cheery manner and wish me a pleasant day. And when he was not in a hurry, as he seemed to always walk with a purpose, he would stop and ask, how I was and what crazy escape from work plan was I conjuring up now? Peter always seemed to be in a good mood, but he would often blame his demeanor on being Irish and how he could not accept any responsibility for actions. Peter was usually often pragmatic in his approach to things, but also fun to be around, and always an optimist, again being Irish and all.

So very sad to have learned of his passing after a good fight with the beast. I will always hold fond memories of Peter, and I am especially grateful for his comments that one day and for him being so blunt in pointing me to the exit door of government. I did it and have never looked back. Thank you Peter.

Kevin. "

I only knew Peter for a short time, but I felt like we knew each other for ages. I think that was just how Peter made people feel once you got to know him- comfortable in his presence and like an old friend. I remember our first real conversation: I set up some time with him and asked him to explain some Yukon lands things (the famous LSA!) and he proceeded to ask me several direct questions about my work and also my life. I guess my answers were acceptable, because he shared his knowledge with me freely from that point on. He also shared his time, kindness, and feelings - which I considered a real privilege. He would often apologize for 'gabbing' so much- but the truth is that I never tired of talking to him, regardless of the subject. Working with him didn't feel like much work, and I wish I had told him. One of the things that I truly admired about Peter, was his ability to do just that: recognize the things he liked about people and tell them. He often used to say how 'awesome' or 'brilliant' he thought I was and I would laugh or make a joke to shrug it off. He stopped me one day and said I really needed to work on taking a compliment. I am working on both of these things and hope to emulate Peter in this regard.

Peter made an impression on me, he impacted me as a person and I am grateful that I got to be one of the people he spent some of his time with.

My thoughts and prayers to his loved ones and everyone else's hearts that he touched.

Heather Kelly

Thank you for your strength and Friendship. I miss you, Peter :: Love Carmen :: Hugs special Carmen hugs to you!! :;

PETER
Even though I never told you, you've been like a father to me. In so many ways, I don't think I needed to tell you in words. You knew.
— Michael

Thank you for being you!
Aaron D.

Peter ...
Noone will *ever* understand
the uniqueness of our shared
experience. You were a
gift to me ... and my family
at a most difficult time.
THANK You for listening.
THANK you for caring.
Your 'chemo buddy'
Joe Iles.

Peter,
You were the most truly
genuine person I have ever
met. You taught me how to be true to
myself. Thankyou my birthday brother. DS

Peter,
To my Kootney
brother I will
miss you... you
are an inspiration.
I love you.
Your Kootney Sister
Ellen.

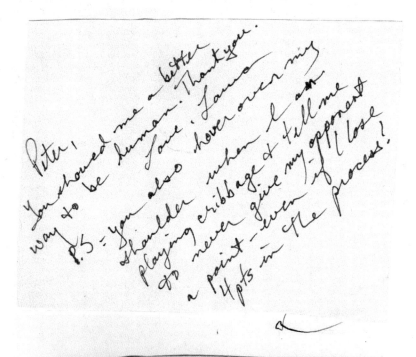

Peter,
You showed me a better
way to be human. Thank you.
Love, Laura
P.S. = you also hover over my
shoulder when I am
playing cribbage & tell me
to never give my opponent
a point - even if I lose
4 pts in the process?

Early Birds at work,
favorite memory is
Peter in sock feet passing
my cubby on the way to the kitchen.
Always a cheerful greeting exchanged!!
♡ Kristen

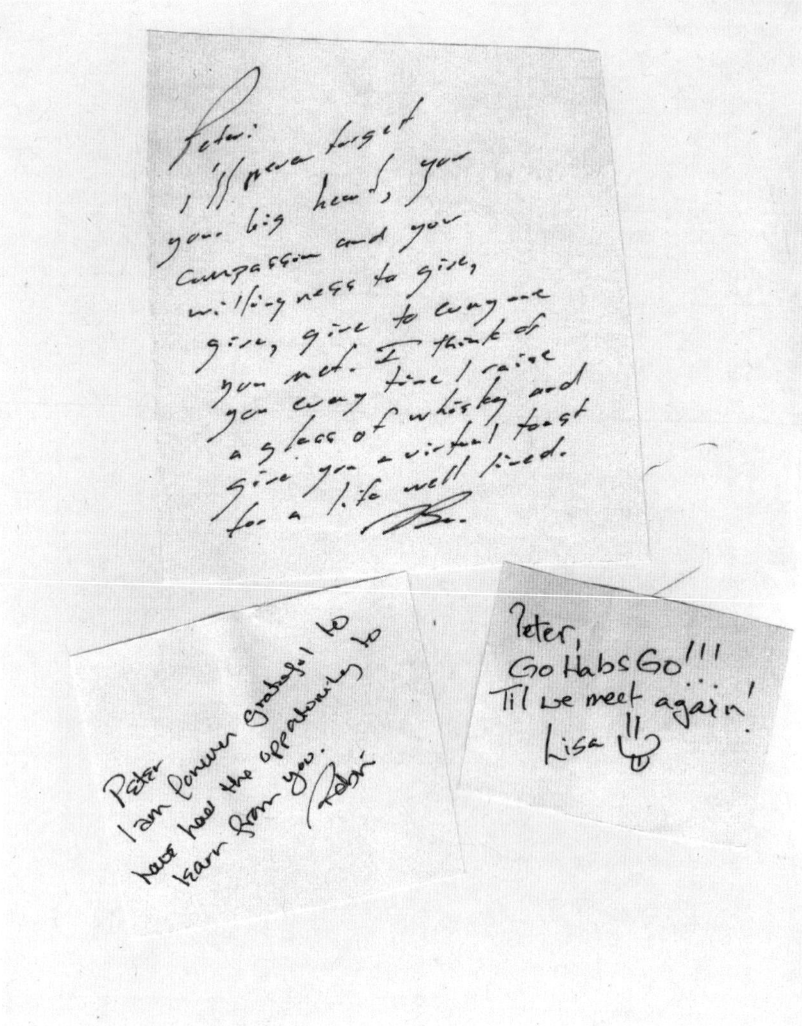

Peter:
I'll never forget
your big heart, your
compassion and your
willingness to give,
give, give to everyone
you met. I think of
you every time I raise
a glass of whisky and
give you a virtual toast
for a life well lived.

Peter
I am forever grateful to
have had the opportunity to
learn from you.
Robin

Peter,
Go Habs Go!!!
Til we meet again!
Lisa